DAY & OVERNIGHT HIKES

Shenandoah

NATIONAL PARK

Other Books by Johnny Molloy

60 Hikes within 60 Miles: Austin &
 San Antonio (with Tom Taylor)
60 Hikes within 60 Miles: Nashville
The Best in Tent Camping: The Carolinas
The Best in Tent Camping: Colorado
The Best in Tent Camping: Florida
The Best in Tent Camping: Georgia
The Best in Tent Camping: Tennessee and Kentucky
The Best in Tent Camping: West Virginia
The Best in Tent Camping: Wisconsin
Day & Overnight Hikes in the
 Great Smoky Mountains National Park
Day & Overnight Hikes in West Virginia's
 Monongahela National Forest
Land Between the Lakes
 Outdoor Recreation Handbook
Long Trails of the Southeast
Mount Rogers
 Outdoor Recreation Handbook

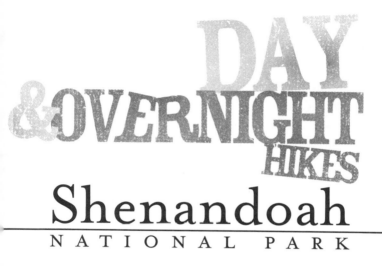

DAY
&OVERNIGHT
HIKES

Shenandoah
NATIONAL PARK

SECOND EDITION

JOHNNY MOLLOY

MENASHA RIDGE PRESS

Published by Menasha Ridge Press
Printed in Canada
Distributed by The Globe Pequot Press
Second edition, first printing

Text and cover design by Ian Szymkowiak (Palace Press
    International)
Cover photograph by Karl Weatherly © Getty Images
Author photograph © Lisa Daniel
Typesetting by Bud Zehmer
Cartography and elevation profiles by Steve Jones & Bud Zehmer

Cataloging-in-Publication Data
Molloy, Johnny, 1961-
Great day and overnight hikes in Shenandoah National Park / by
Johnny Molloy.-2nd ed
p.   cm.
Includes index.
ISBN 0-89732-526-5

1. Hiking—Virginia—Shenandoah National Park—
Guidebooks.2. Backpacking—Shenandoah National Park—
Guidebooks.3. Shenandoah National Park—Guidebooks. I
Title.

GV199.42.V82S4846 2003
917.55'90444—dc21   2003051319
                                     CIP

Menasha Ridge Press
P.O. Box 43673
Birmingham, Alabama 35243
www.menasharidge.com

Table of Contents

Part I: Great Out and Backs

THE NORTH DISTRICT

THE CENTRAL DISTRICT

THE SOUTH DISTRICT

Part II: Great Day Loops

Part III: Great Overnight Loops

Dedication

This book is for Christy Crutchfield, an enduring and endearing friend.

Acknowledgments

I would like to thank the following people for their help in creating this book: Shenandoah National Park Rangers Steve Bair, Matt Richardson, and David Bauer; Andrea, Cara, and Lisa at Shenandoah River Outfitters; Robin and Anna from Overall Run; Karen Michaud, Emily Holcomb, Bud Zehmer, Katie Woychak, Sofie Grayson, Hunt Cochrane, Francisco Meyer, Keny Slay, Janet Wuethrich, and especially David Zaczyk. Everyone made this an enjoyable and rewarding project.

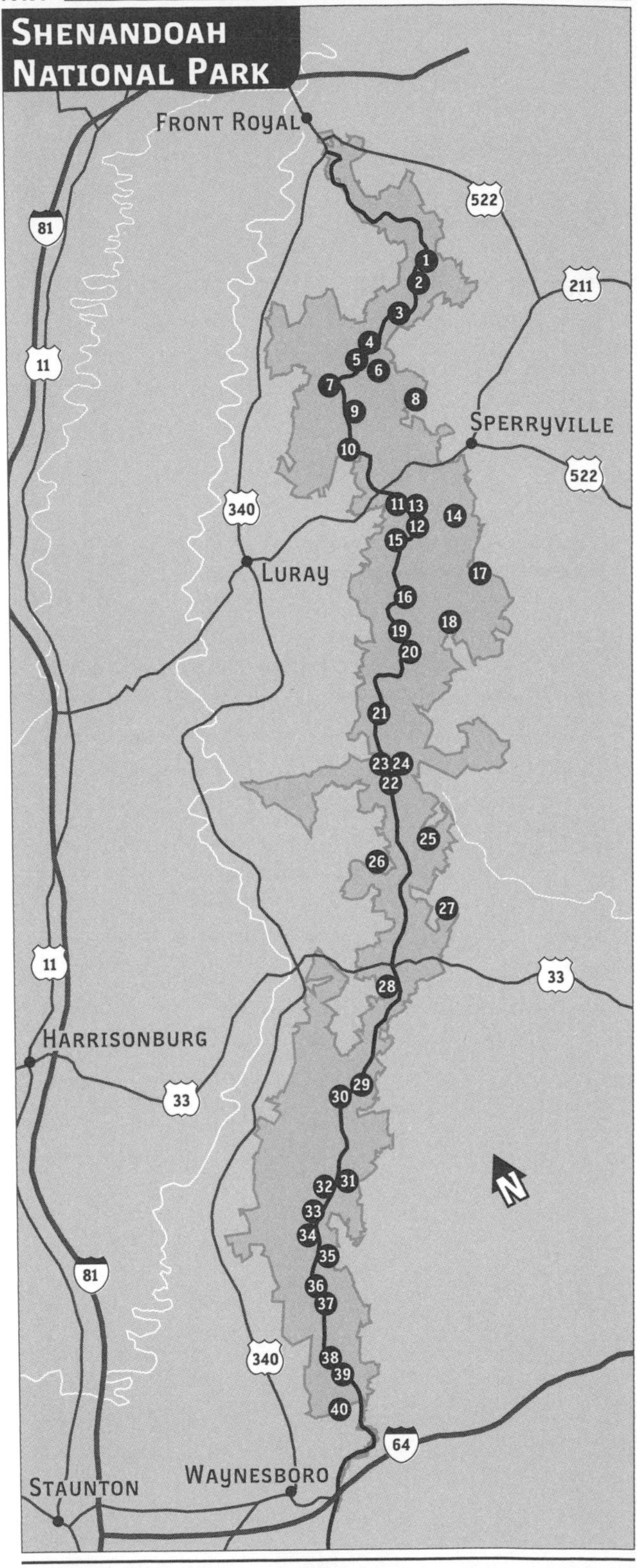

SHENANDOAH NATIONAL PARK

FRONT ROYAL

81

522

11

211

1
2
3
4
5
6
7
8
9
10

SPERRYVILLE

340

522

11
12
13
14
15
16
17
18
19
20

LURAY

21

23 24
22

25

26

27

28

33

HARRISONBURG

33

29
30 31
32
33
34
35
36 37
38
39
40

11

81

340

64

STAUNTON

WAYNESBORO

Map Key

Preface

SHENANDOAH NATIONAL PARK is the scenic mountain haven of the eastern seaboard. The park offers panoramic views from overlooks scattered on lofty Skyline Drive, which runs the length of the 300-square-mile sanctuary. Beyond Skyline Drive lies another Shenandoah, where bears furtively roam the hollows and brook trout ply the tumbling streams. Quartz, granite, and greenstone outcrops jut above the diverse forest, allowing far-flung views of the Blue Ridge and surrounding Shenandoah Valley.

You must reach this other Shenandoah by foot. The rewards increase with every footfall beneath the stately oaks of the ridge tops and in the deep canyons where waterfalls roar among old-growth trees spared by the logger's axe. In some places your footsteps will lead you past pioneer cemeteries. The gravestones reveal another era of Shenandoah. It is a rich cultural history that once found pioneer farms squeezed into the narrow valleys and apple orchards lining grassy fields atop the ridges, where lives were lived in the shadows of these Appalachian highlands.

This meld of natural and cultural history is fitting in Virginia, where so much of this country's story has been played out, from the battles of the American Revolutionary and Civil War to battles in Congress where this park was established. Shenandoah National Park has also seen the depopulation and reforestation of the park, the building of Skyline Drive, the return of the deer, and the invasion of exotic pests that threaten the mountain trees. And through it all, Shenandoah has shone.

Shenandoah National Park offers much to see, yet our hurried lives afford little time to see it all. However, a respite in the mountains will revitalize both mind and spirit. Smell the autumn leaves on a crisp afternoon. Climb to a lookout. Contemplate pioneer lives at an old homesite. Put your life into perspective.

That is where this book will come into play. It will help you make every step count, whether you are leading the family on a brief day hike or undertaking a challenging backpack into the remote reaches of the park. With the knowledge you find here, your outdoor experience and your precious time can be utilized to its fullest.

Often, park sightseers randomly pick a hike without knowing where it will lead, or they follow the crowds wherever they go. Many times, I've been stopped with the question, "What's down this trail?" Choosing a hike at random in Shenandoah, where many trails drop steeply off the Blue Ridge, may result in a rigorous return to the car with no rewards to show effort.

This book presents more than 30 day hikes from which to choose. Classic hikes, such as Old Rag and Whiteoak Canyon, are included. However, though the majority of these hikes are not as well known, they offer as much solitude and equally scenic sights—like Big Branch Falls and Furnace Mountain—as the more popular hikes. This will give you the opportunity to get back to nature on your own terms.

Two types of day hikes are offered: one-way and loop hikes. One-way hikes lead to a particularly rewarding destination and return via the same trail. The return trip allows you to see everything from the opposite vantage point. You may notice more minute trailside features the second go-round, and returning at a different time of day may give the same trail a surprisingly different character. But to some, returning on the same trail just isn't enjoyable. Some hikers just can't stand the thought of covering the same ground twice with 500 other miles of Shenandoah trails awaiting them. The loop hikes provide an alternative.

Most of the hikes offer solitude to maximize your Shenandoah experience, although portions of some hikes traverse potentially popular areas. It should also be noted that loop hikes are generally longer and harder than one-way hikes, but a bigger challenge can reap bigger rewards.

Day hiking is the best and most popular way to "break into" the Shenandoah wilderness. But for those with the inclination to see the mountain cycle from day to night and back again, this book offers ten overnight hikes with the best locales for camping. The length of these hikes—three days and two nights—was chosen primarily for the weekend backpacker. Backpackers must follow park regulations and practice "leave no trace" wilderness-use etiquette.

When touring Shenandoah, it's a great temptation to remain in your car and enjoy the sights along Skyline Drive. While auto touring is a great way to get an overview of the park, it creates a barrier between you and the wilderness beyond. Windshield tourists hoping to observe wildlife often end up observing only the traffic around them. While overlooks avail easy views, the hassle of driving, the drone of traffic, and the lack of effort in reaching the views can make them less than inspirational. Shenandoah is great for hiking.

The wilderness experience can unleash your mind and body allowing you to relax and find peace and quiet. It also enables you to grasp beauty and splendor: a white-quartz outcrop with a window overlooking the patchwork valley below, a bobcat disappearing into a laurel thicket, or a snow-covered clearing marking an old homestead. On these protected lands you can let your mind roam free to go where it pleases. This simply can't be achieved in a climate-controlled automobile.

The following sections offer advice on how to use this book and how to have a safe and pleasant hike in the woods. Shenandoah is a special preserve; get out and enjoy it.

– Johnny Molloy

Introduction

━━ How to Use This Guidebook

At the top of the section for each hike is a box
that allows the hiker quick access to pertinent information: quality of scenery, difficulty of hike,
condition of trail, quality of solitude expected,
appropriateness for children, distance, approxi-
mate time of hike, and highlights of the trip.
The first five categories are rated using a five-star
system. Below is an example of a box included
with a hike:

Broad Hollow *Pine Hill Gap Loop*

Scenery:✰ ✰ ✰ ✰ ✰
Trail Condition:✰ ✰ ✰
Children: ✰ ✰
Difficulty: ✰ ✰
Solitude: ✰ ✰ ✰
Distance: *3.4 miles round-trip*
Hiking time: *2:45 round-trip*
Outstanding Features: *Wide-ranging views from two vista points*

The five stars indicate the scenery is very picturesque. The two stars indicate it is a relatively
easy hike (five stars for difficulty would be stren-
uous). The trail condition is fairly good (one
star would mean the trail is likely to be muddy,
rocky, overgrown, or have some obstacle). You
can expect to encounter only a few people on the
trail (with one star you may well be elbowing your
way up the trail). And the hike is doable for able-
bodied children (a one-star rating would denote
that only the most gung ho and physically fit
children should go).

Distances given are absolute, but hiking
times are estimated for the average hiker making
a round-trip. Overnight-hiking times account
for the burden of carrying a pack.

Following each box is a brief description of the hike. A more detailed account follows, in which trail junctions, stream crossings, and trailside features are noted along with their distance from the trailhead. This should help you keep apprised of your whereabouts as well as ensure that you don't miss those features noted. You can use this guidebook to walk just a portion of a hike or to plan a hike of your own by combining the information.

The hikes have been divided into one-way day hikes, loop day hikes, and overnight loop hikes. Each type of hike is separated by the park district in which it lies: either north, central, or south. These districts are divided by prominent gaps in the park through which roads pass to allow easier access from the surrounding lowlands. Feel free to flip through the book, read the descriptions, and choose a hike that appeals to you.

Weather

Each of the four distinct seasons lays its hands on Shenandoah National Park, though elevation always factors into park weather patterns. While each season brings exciting changes in the flora and fauna, the changes can occur seemingly day-to-day rather than month-to-month.

Be prepared for a wide range of temperatures and conditions regardless of the season. As a rule of thumb, the temperature decreases about three degrees for every 1,000 feet of elevation gained. The approximately 50 inches of yearly precipitation on the Blue Ridge is about 15 inches more than the nearby Shenandoah Valley receives. This precipitation is evenly distributed throughout the year, though it arrives with slow-moving frontal systems in winter and with thunderstorms in summer.

Spring is the most variable season. During March, you'll find the first signs of rebirth in the lowlands, yet trees in the high country may not be fully leafed out until June. Both winter- and summer-like weather can be experienced in spring. As summer approaches, the weather warms, the strong fronts weaken, and thunderstorms and haze become more frequent. Summertime rainy days can be cool. In fall, continental fronts once again sweep through, clearing the air and bringing warm days and cool nights, though rain is always possible.

The first snow of winter usually arrives in November, and snow can intermittently fall through April, though no permanent snowpack exists. About 40 inches of snow will fall during this time. Expect to incur entire days of below-freezing weather, though temperatures can range from mild to bitterly cold.

Clothing

There is a wide variety of clothing from which to choose. Basically, use common sense and be prepared for anything. If all you have are cotton clothes when a sudden rainstorm comes along, you'll be miserable, especially in cooler weather. It's a good idea to carry along a light wool sweater or some type of synthetic apparel (polypropylene, Capeline, Thermax, etc.) as well as a hat.

Always carry raingear. Thunderstorms can come on suddenly in the summer, and winter fronts can soak you to the bone. Keep in mind that rainy days are as much a part of nature as those idyllic ones you desire. Besides, rainy days really cut down on the crowds. With appropriate raingear, a normally crowded trail can be a wonderful place of solitude. Do, however, remember that getting wet opens the door to hypothermia.

Footwear is another concern. Though tennis shoes may be appropriate for paved areas, many Shenandoah trails are rocky and rough; tennis shoes may not offer enough support. Waterproofed or not, boots should be your footwear of choice. Sport sandals are more popular than ever, but these leave much of your foot exposed. An injured foot far from the trailhead can make for a miserable limp back to the car.

To some potential mountain enthusiasts, the deep woods seem inordinately dark and perilous. It is the fear of the unknown that causes this anxiety. No doubt, potentially dangerous situations can occur outdoors, but as long as you use sound judgment and prepare yourself before hitting the trail, you'll be much safer in the woods than in most urban areas of the country. It is better to look at a backcountry hike as a fascinating chance to discover the unknown rather than a chance for potential disaster. Here are a few tips to make your trip safer and easier.

• Always carry food and water whether you are planning to go overnight or not. Food will give you energy, help keep you warm, and sustain you in an emergency situation until help arrives. You never know if you will have a stream nearby when you become thirsty. Bring potable water or treat water before drinking it from a stream. The chance of getting sick from the organism known as giardia or other waterborne organisms is small, but there is no reason to take that chance. Boil or filter all water before drinking it.

• Stay on designated trails. Most hikers get lost when they leave the path. If you become disoriented, don't panic—that may result in a bad decision that will make your predicament worse. Retrace your steps if you can remember them or stay where you are. Rangers check the trails first when searching for lost or overdue hikers. Though remaining in one place is the best option, you may choose to follow a creek or drainage downstream; because Shenandoah is a long, narrow park, this should eventually lead you to the civilized world.

• Take a map, compass, and lighter, and know how to use them. Should you become lost, these three items can keep you around long enough to be found or get you out of a pickle. A compass can help you orient yourself, and a lighter can start a fire for signaling help and keeping warm. Trail maps are available at entrance stations or visitor centers.

• Be especially careful when crossing streams. Whether you are fording the stream or crossing on a log, make every step count. If you have any doubt about maintaining your balance on a foot log, go ahead and ford the stream instead. When fording a stream, use a stout tree limb or cane for balance and face upstream as you cross. If a stream seems too deep to ford, turn back. Whatever is on the other side is not worth risking your life.

• Be careful at overlooks. Shenandoah has numerous bluffs and outcrops. While these areas may provide spectacular views, they are potentially hazardous. Stay back from the edge of outcrops and be absolutely sure of your footing; a misstep can mean a nasty and possibly fatal fall.

• Standing dead trees and storm-damaged living trees pose a real hazard to hikers. These trees may have loose or broken limbs that could fall at any time. When choosing a spot to rest or a backcountry campsite, look up.

• Know the symptoms of hypothermia. Shivering and forgetfulness are the two most common indicators of this cold-weather killer. Hypothermia can occur at higher elevations, even in the summer, especially when the hiker is wearing lightweight cotton clothing. If symptoms arise, get the victim shelter, hot liquids, and dry clothes or a dry sleeping bag.

• Avoid bear-fear paralysis. The black bears of Shenandoah are wild animals, hence they are unpredictable. If you see one, give it a wide berth and don't feed it, and you'll be fine. There has never been a recorded death caused by a bear in Shenandoah; most injuries have occurred when an ignorant visitor fed or otherwise harassed a wild bear. So don't stay in your car for fear of bears, just give them plenty of respect.

• Take along your brain. A cool, calculating mind is the single most important piece of equipment you'll ever need on the trail. Think before you act. Watch your step. Plan ahead. Avoiding accidents before they happen is the best recipe for a rewarding and relaxing hike.

• Ask questions. Park employees are there to help. It's a lot easier to gain advice beforehand and avoid a mishap away from civilization when it's too late to amend an error. Use your head out there and treat the place as if it were your own backyard. After all, it is your national park.

Tips for Enjoying Shenandoah National Park

Before you go, call the national park for an information kit; call (540) 999-3500. This will help you get oriented to Shenandoah's roads, features, and attractions. Detailed maps of the three park districts are available through the Shenandoah Natural History Association; call (540) 999-3582. They will really help you get around the park's backcountry. In addition, the following tips will make your visit enjoyable and more rewarding.

• Get out of your car and onto a trail. Auto touring allows a cursory overview of the park, but only from a visual perspective. On the trail you can use your ears and nose as well. This guidebook recommends some trails over others, but any trail is better than no trail at all.

• Investigate different areas of the park. The Appalachian Trail links the three park districts. The South District is very rocky with white-quartz outcrops. Many waterfalls tumble throughout the Central District. The North District is rich in human history and wildlife. A mosaic of forests covers Shenandoah entirety. You'll be pleasantly surprised to see so many distinct landscapes in one national park.

• Take your time along the trails. Pace yourself. Shenandoah is filled with wonders both big and small. Don't rush past a tiny salamander to get to that overlook. Stop and smell the wildflowers. Peer into a clear mountain stream to find brook trout. Don't miss the trees for the forest.

• We can't always schedule our free time when we want, but try to hike during the week and avoid the traditional holidays if possible. Trails that are packed in the summer are often clear during the colder months. If you are hiking on a busy day, go early in the morning; it'll enhance your chances of seeing wildlife. The trails really clear out during rainy times, however, don't hike during a thunderstorm.

BACKCOUNTRY ADVICE

BE SURE TO GET THE REQUIRED (but free) backcountry-camping permit before you embark on your overnight trip. You can get a permit in person at entrance stations, visitor centers, park headquarters, and some self-registration stations, or call (540) 999-3500 to receive a mailed permit. Regulations change occasionally, so be sure to ask about the current regulations when you get a permit. At press time, the following regulations were active.

You can camp anywhere in the park with the following restrictions: when possible, use pre-existing campsites that are at least 20 yards from trails and unpaved roads; you may use a pristine site if no existing site is available; camp at least 10 yards from any water sources; camp one-quarter mile from any developed areas and the Skyline Drive.

Solid human waste must be buried in a hole at least three inches deep and at least 20 yards away from trails and water sources; a trowel is basic backpacking equipment. Otherwise, "Pack it in, pack it out." Practice "leave no trace" camping ethics while in the backcountry. An informational handout on "leave no trace" ethics is available wherever you obtain your permit.

Open fires are not permitted except at some Appalachian Trail huts; backpacking stoves are strongly encouraged. Please do not take glass containers into the backcountry. You are required to hang your food from bears and other animals in order to minimize human impact on wildlife and to avoid their introduction to and dependence on human food. Wildlife learns to associate backpacks and backpackers with easy food sources, thereby influencing their behavior. Make sure you have about 30 feet of rope to properly secure your food. Ideally you should throw your rope over a stout limb that extends 10 or more feet above ground. Make sure the rope hangs at least 5 feet away from the tree trunk.

It may seem a backcountry trip is fraught with rules and regulations, but the whole scheme is designed for a pleasant, safe, low-impact interaction between man and nature. The rules are intended to enhance your experience within the confines of this Blue Ridge refuge. Note that park regulations can change over time; contact the park to confirm the status of the above regulations before you enter the backcountry.

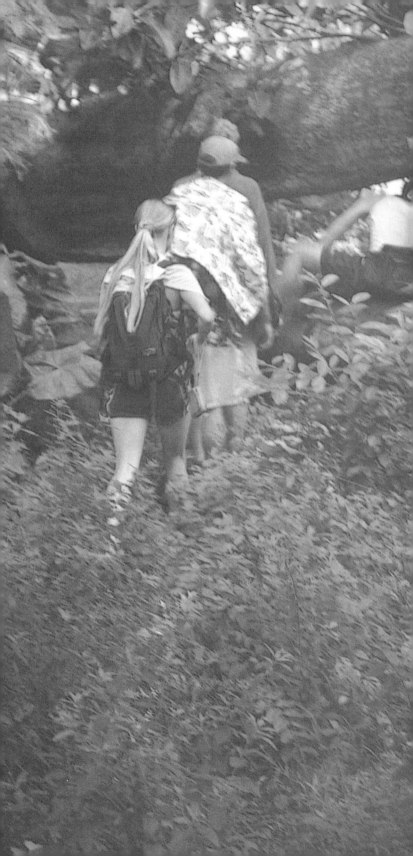

The return trip to the AT will get you huffing and puffing, while thinking of all the people that skipped this second view as is evidenced by the much less used trail tread.

Compton Peak *from Jenkins Gap*

SCENERY: ✿ ✿ ✿ ✿ ✿
TRAIL CONDITION: ✿ ✿ ✿
CHILDREN: ✿ ✿
DIFFICULTY: ✿ ✿
SOLITUDE: ✿ ✿
DISTANCE: *3.4 miles round-trip*
HIKING TIME: *2:45 round-trip*
OUTSTANDING FEATURES: *wide-ranging views from two vista points*

THIS OUT-AND-BACK DAY HIKE *takes the lesser-used approach to a mountaintop with two good vistas from rock protrusions along its flanks. The Appalachian Trail (AT) is your host along the way to these two outcrops. For a climb to a vista, this isn't too steep.*

🕺 Begin this walk on the Jenkins Gap Trail. The yellow-blazed pathway leaves from the parking area around auto-blocking boulders to intersect the AT in 150 feet. Turn right, heading northbound on the AT. The walking is easy in a mixed forest of sugar maple, cherry, locust, and ever-present oak shading a brushy forest floor. Keep a level track through the actual Jenkins Gap. Skyline Drive is to your right. After a while you begin to wonder about the climb to Compton Peak. Finally, after 0.5 miles, the trail veers left and ascends a mountainside of chestnut oak and mountain laurel.

Switchback on some elaborate stone steps built during a trail reroute. Step over a little spring branch at 0.9 miles and look for apple trees persisting in the forest beyond the spring. These are remnants of an orchard on the north and south side of Jenkins Gap.

Reach a four-way trail junction at mile 1.3. Your vista choices go left or right. Head left on the blue-blazed trail, to the more popular and widespread view. Briefly continue climbing over a rock knob before dipping to an outcrop with a widespread vista at 1.5 miles. Below, the path of Skyline Drive is evident as it snakes downhill along Dickey Ridge. To the far left are the South Fork of the Shenandoah River and the Shenandoah Valley. Ahead, more mountains and the flatlands extend toward Washington, D.C. This is a truly inspiring vista.

The second vista is more challenging to reach. If you have made it this far, go ahead and check out the

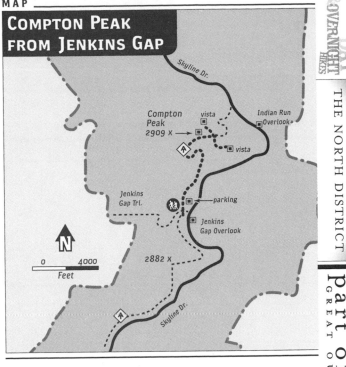

COMPTON PEAK
FROM JENKINS GAP

Skyline Dr.

Compton
Peak
2909 X →

vista

Indian Run
Overlook

vista

Jenkins
Gap Trl.

parking

Jenkins
Gap Overlook

N

0   4000
Feet

2882 X

Skyline Dr.

ELEVATION PROFILE

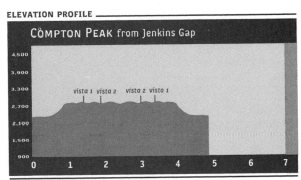

CÒMPTON PEAK from Jenkins Gap

4,500
3,900
3,300
2,700
2,100
1,500
900

vista 1 vista 2   vista 2 vista 1

0   1   2   3   4   5   6   7

second view. Backtrack to reach the AT and keep forward, now on the second blue-blazed path. The trail
is more faint as it goes down, down, down on a rocky
tread. Reach an outcrop where you might expect a
vista, but keep hiking. Hike down the bluff, walk a
few feet through the woods and scramble up a rocky
prominence at mile 1.9. This prominence offers
worthy views of Mount Marshall in the foreground
and lands east of the Blue Ridge. While thinking of
the unfortunate people who skip this second view, as
evidenced by its less-used trail, the return trip to the
AT will get you huffing and puffing.

Big Devils Stairs

SCENERY: ✩ ✩ ✩ ✩ ✩
DIFFICULTY: ✩ ✩
TRAIL CONDITION: ✩ ✩ ✩ ✩
SOLITUDE: ✩ ✩ ✩
CHILDREN: ✩ ✩ ✩
DISTANCE: *5.4 miles round-trip*
HIKING TIME: *3:15 round-trip*
OUTSTANDING FEATURES: *great views, easy hiking, Appalachian Trail hut*

THIS IS A MODERATE HIKE *with a great reward. The walking is easy, and the trails are used surprisingly little. The nearly level Bluff Trail takes you to the Big Devils Stairs canyon rim for a great view of the valley below and the mountains beyond. Along the way, you will pass a shelter used by long-distance hikers on the Appalachian Trail.*

🚶🚶 Leave Skyline Drive from the rear of the Gravel Springs Gap parking area on the Appalachian Trail. Head south for 0.1 mile and turn left on the Bluff Trail. Switchback 0.3 miles down through a dense forest to emerge at the Gravel Springs Hut. In front of you is the spring and to your right is the trail shelter. Imagine staying in shelters like this on the 2,100-mile trek from Georgia to Maine.

This hike continues on the Bluff Trail, which leaves the clearing from the shelter on the right. At the Harris Hollow Trail junction, continue forward on the Bluff Trail. After a switchback, come to another junction; stay left and continue on the Bluff Trail. It runs nearly level, around 2,300 feet, on the southeast slope of Mount Marshall beneath a high-canopied forest strewn with large boulders.

At 1.1 miles, the forest opens on the right, offering views from the side of Mount Marshall. Several of Gravel Springs branches emanate from the slopes of Mount Marshall and bisect the Bluff Trail. Many of these will be dry in late summer and fall.

At mile 1.9, cross the upper reaches of Big Devils Stairs gorge, which is just beginning to cut its way

BIG DEVILS STAIRS

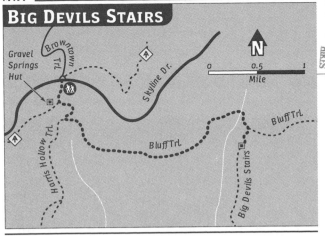

Gravel Springs Hut

Browntown Trl

Skyline Dr.

N

0   0.5   1
Mile

Harris Hollow Trl.

Bluff Trl.

Bluff Trl.

Big Devils Stairs

ELEVATION PROFILE

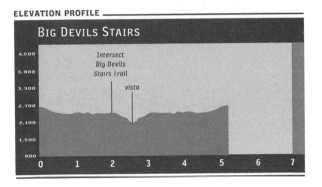

BIG DEVILS STAIRS

Intersect
Big Devils
Stairs Trail

vista

4,500
3,900
3,300
2,700
2,100
1,500
900

0   1   2   3   4   5   6   7

down the mountainside. It is an easy crossing in times of normal water flow. Just beyond the crossing, come to the Big Devils Stairs Trail junction.

Turn right onto the Big Devils Stairs Trail, which follows the east rim of the gorge. Notice how the forest changes. The trees here are those typically found on drier slopes—chestnut oak and Virginia pine—with an understory of mountain laurel. At mile 2.2, the path makes a few switchbacks as it meanders down the rim of the gorge.

After an abrupt right turn, the trail comes to the edge of the gorge, offering a southward view. Continue down the trail and descend to a large rock outcrop at mile 2.6. There are good views of the Big Devils Stairs canyon and the mountains beyond. Follow the trail just 0.1 mile farther to another outcrop that hosts a gnarled pine hanging on the edge of the rim. Here there are even better views of the beautiful Shenandoah country. Beyond this point, the trail begins a steep descent and is not recommended.

DIRECTIONS: From Thornton Gap, take Skyline Drive
north for 13.9 miles to the Gravel Springs Gap parking area
at milepost 17.6. It is on the right side of Skyline Drive. The
Appalachian Trail leaves the rear of the parking area.

Overall Run Falls

SCENERY: ☆ ☆ ☆ ☆ ☆
DIFFICULTY: ☆ ☆
TRAIL CONDITION: ☆ ☆ ☆ ☆
SOLITUDE: ☆
CHILDREN: ☆ ☆ ☆
DISTANCE: *6.4 miles round-trip*
HIKING TIME: *4:00 round-trip*
OUTSTANDING FEATURES: *highest falls in park, great view*

THIS OUT-AND-BACK HIKE HOLDS *a great reward when you
arrive at its far end. And the hike is not too hard, either. Start with a
pleasant mountaintop stroll, and make your way down the slopes of
Hogback Mountain, entering the Overall Run watershed. Pass a
warm-up falls then arrive at Overall Run Falls. From a rocky
precipice you can see the nearby cataract against a background of
valley and mountains. Others will be enjoying the scenery with you.*

🏃 Pick up the Appalachian Trail (AT) as it skirts
the south side of the Hogback Mountain Overlook
parking area. Turn right onto the AT, heading
south. Gently climb through a fern-carpeted woodland, passing a few rock outcrops. Level off, then
turn right on the Tuscarora-Overall Run Trail at 0.4
miles. The trail wends its way between rocks, making
a couple of switchbacks before reaching another trail
junction at 1.1 mile.

Turn right, staying on the Tuscarora–Overall
Run Trail. Pass a large embedded rock on your left,
then begin making your way down Hogback
Mountain in stair-step fashion. The path will drop,
level off, drop again, and level off once more.
Continue in this pattern, passing a couple of wet-
weather draws, and end up in the Overall Run watershed. Here the trail intersects the Mathews Arm Trail
at mile 2.7.

Keep going forward. Both trails run a short distance along the same path before the Mathews Arm
Trail veers off to the right. The Tuscarora–Overall
Run Trail turns and heads down to Overall Run,
coming to some falls at mile 2.9. A side trail leads

OVERALL RUN FALLS

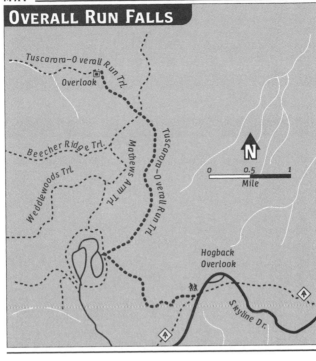

ELEVATION PROFILE

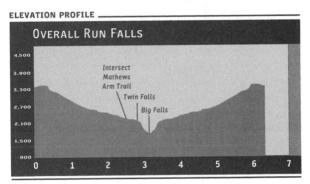

OVERALL RUN FALLS

left to the top of this waterfall. Here Overall Run is split by a large boulder, forcing the creek to divide, resulting in 2 streams dropping 29 feet. This is only the warm-up falls.

Continue along the side of the canyon, descending again. Come to a cliff at mile 3.2, where the world opens before you. To your left is Overall Run Falls, dropping over sheer rock into the gorge below (at 93 feet it is the park's highest). Beyond you is Overall Run canyon, which opens up to Page Valley and Massanutten Mountain. In the distance are the Alleghenies. A great view, overall.

DIRECTIONS: From Thornton Gap, take Skyline Drive
north for 10.4 miles to the parking area just before Hogback
Mountain Overlook. It will be on your left at milepost 21.1.
You can park at Hogback Overlook and walk the short distance to where the AT passes directly by the south end of the
parking area. Turn right and head southbound on the AT.

Piney River Falls

SCENERY: ✿ ✿ ✿ ✿
DIFFICULTY: ✿ ✿
TRAIL CONDITION: ✿ ✿ ✿
SOLITUDE: ✿ ✿ ✿ ✿
CHILDREN: ✿ ✿ ✿
DISTANCE: *6.8 miles round-trip*
HIKING TIME: *4:45 round-trip*
OUTSTANDING FEATURES: *Piney River Falls, isolation*

IT'S SURPRISING THAT THIS HIKE ISN'T *more popular. The
scenery along the way meets high Shenandoah standards, and the
falls are a worthy destination. To get there, leave the Piney River
Developed Area and gently wind your way through an eye-pleasing,
high-country woods. Work your way down through the Piney River
valley on old roads and take a short side trail to the three-tiered
falls. It's a good way to spend an afternoon.*

    Start your hike at the back of the field between
Skyline Drive and the parking area across from the old
CCC camp building (now used as a maintenance
office). Look for the concrete post marked "Piney
Branch Trail." Begin walking through a forest of black
locust trees that are in the process of taking over a
field. At 0.1 mile intersect the Appalachian Trail (AT)
and continue forward, crossing a grassy lane.

    The Piney Branch Trail winds its way down to the
valley, making very gentle switchbacks. It comes to
the upper reaches of the Piney River at mile 1.3 and
curves right to cross more feeder streams. The trail
arrives at the junction with the Pole Bridge Link
Trail at mile 1.4.

    Turn right and stay on the Piney Branch Trail.
The path follows an old road on a slight downgrade.
Notice the gorge of Piney River on your right. At
mile 2, the old road continues forward, but the
Piney Branch Trail veers right and follows another
old road. The trail runs a fair distance above the
creek, descending at a moderate but steady clip.

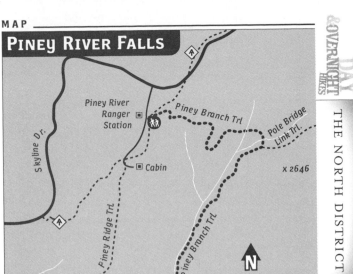

ELEVATION PROFILE

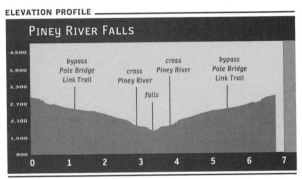

Cross the Piney River at mile 3. You are now on the western side of the river, and the falls are only 0.4 miles away. There are many small cascades along Piney River as you make your way downstream. The forest of the river valley is cove hardwood: basswood, yellow birch, red maple, and hemlock, which, in the eastern U.S., has fallen prey to the woolly adelgid.

Pass two house-sized rock bluffs on your right at mile 3.2. Begin listening for the falls, which are only 0.2 miles away. At mile 3.4, turn left on a side trail leading to the Falls. Piney River Falls is a 25-foot, 3-tiered cascade that flows over mossy rock into a deep and wide pool. It's a good place to cool off after a hot hike. Be careful getting to and from the falls.

> **DIRECTIONS:** From Thornton Gap, take Skyline Drive north for 9.4 miles to Piney River Developed Area. The entrance road is on your right at milepost 22.1, just after you pass the turn to Mathews Arm Campground on the left. Park in the designated visitor parking area. The Piney Branch Trail starts between the parking area and Skyline Drive.

Hazel Falls

SCENERY: ☆ ☆ ☆ ☆
DIFFICULTY: ☆ ☆
TRAIL CONDITION: ☆ ☆ ☆ ☆
SOLITUDE: ☆ ☆ ☆
CHILDREN: ☆ ☆ ☆ ☆
DISTANCE: *5.2 miles round-trip*
HIKING TIME: *3:00 round-trip*
OUTSTANDING FEATURES: *waterfall, rock "cave"*

THIS HIKE TAKES YOU INTO "HAZEL COUNTRY," *a heavily settled area in pre-park days. The route traverses varied terrain and drops down to the Hazel River, where a small rock indentation forms a natural shelter beside a waterfall. All in all, it's a good destination.*

🚶 The difficulty of this hike is hard to rate: the first 2.3-mile portion is a gentle stroll on old roads, but the last 0.3-mile trek to the cave and falls is on a steep, rough footpath. Though rugged, this section is short; all but the smallest children should make it easily.

Leave Skyline Drive on the Hazel Mountain Fire Road. Descend past a clearing at 0.3 miles and come to a trail junction at 0.5 miles. Veer right on the Hazel Mountain Trail. Hemlock and striped maple crowd the path and form a dense canopy overhead. Soon the trail bears left, levels out, and crosses several small spring branches coming in from the left. In some places, the forest is nearly devoid of ground cover, revealing the spindly trunks of second-growth trees.

The trail sidles alongside the Hazel River at mile 1. "No Camping" signs are posted in the woods nearby. Continue along the river and turn left on the White Rocks Trail at mile 1.6. The path ascends slightly, then

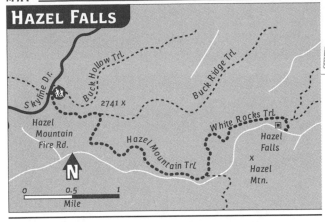

ELEVATION PROFILE

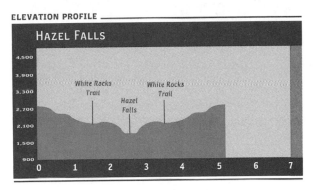

levels out along an old road. Other old roads veer off this trail, but the main path is evident. Large boulders are strewn about the forest, which changes to pine and chestnut oak as the trail tops out on the ridge.

After the trail becomes rockier and descends somewhat, come to an unmarked junction at mile 2.3. The main trail continues forward, while an unmarked footpath veers right. Follow the unmarked footpath downhill. Immediately pass another "No Camping" sign. The trail then drops steeply down an eroded rocky path. Carefully descend to the river. Across the way is Hazel Mountain.

Reach the river at 2.5 miles. Notice the peeling trunks of the many yellow birch. Turn right, following the footpath 0.5 miles upstream to a waterfall. The rock indentation lies on your right at the base of a huge, granite bluff (quite a sturdy roof). It is about 10 feet deep, 30 feet wide, and 8 feet high. The waterfall drops about 30 feet down a narrow chute into a deep pool. The rock notch makes this a good rainy-day destination.

DIRECTIONS: From Thornton Gap, take Skyline Drive
south for 2 miles to the Meadow Spring parking area at
milepost 33.5. The parking area is on the left side of
Skyline Drive.

Marys Rock

SCENERY: ☆ ☆ ☆ ☆ ☆
DIFFICULTY: ☆ ☆
TRAIL CONDITION: ☆ ☆ ☆
SOLITUDE: ☆ ☆ ☆
CHILDREN: ☆ ☆
DISTANCE: *6.8 miles round-trip*
HIKING TIME: *4:00 round-trip*
OUTSTANDING FEATURE: *many outstanding views*

THE HIKE OVER THE PINNACLE TO MARYS ROCK *traverses the
most spectacular section of the Appalachian Trail (AT) through
Shenandoah National Park. The views are expansive and frequent.
And hiking to a view is always more rewarding than driving to a
view. Views open up shortly after you leave Jewell Hollow
Overlook. The Pinnacle is outstanding and many Shenandoah
old-timers feel Marys Rock is the best vista in the entire park. Take
this hike and find out for yourself.*

🕯 Leave from the back of the Jewell Hollow
Overlook and hike 50 feet to the AT. Turn right,
northbound on the AT. The path actually goes south
a short distance before making a switchback to head
north. Come to a small field at 0.2 miles. Enjoy
your first view opening to the west. Begin to climb
beyond the meadow, coming to a trail junction at
0.3 miles. Pass the Leading Ridge Trail and continue
north on the AT.

The path tunnels through an understory of
mountain laurel in dense woodland. At 0.7 miles
enter a forest area littered with massive gray boulders. Meander amid the boulders and reach The
Pinnacle (3,730 feet) at mile 1. Step out on the rock
outcrop and be prepared for an incredible view of
the Virginia mountains and valleys to the west. But
be careful on these jagged, uneven rocks.

The AT continues north and begins to descend
as a series of switchbacks as it nears Byrds Nest
Shelter No. 3 at mile 2. This stone structure has a
picnic table and provides a respite from the ele-

Marys Rock

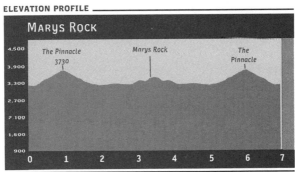

Marys Rock

Meadow
Spring Trl.

Skyline Dr.

x 2775

Buck Hollow Trl

Byrds
Nest

Buck Ridge Trl.

Leading Ridge Trl.

Jewell
Hollow
Overlook

The Pinnacle
3730 x

Skyline Dr.

N

0   0.5   1
Mile

ELEVATION PROFILE

Marys Rock

The Pinnacle
3730

Marys Rock

The
Pinnacle

4,500
3,900
3,300
2,700
2,100
1,500
900
0   1   2   3   4   5   6   7

ments, but don't expect the water fountain to work.
Follow the service road that leads from Byrds Nest to
Skyline Drive for a short distance and veer left, stay-
ing on the AT, which continues at a slight incline.

Another westward view opens at mile 2.4, soon
after a switchback to the left. A rock promontory
offers more views at mile 2.6. Pass the Meadow
Spring Trail at mile 2.8 and begin climbing for 0.3
miles. The trail levels as it approaches the backside of
Marys Rock. Continue downhill to the Marys Rock
spur trail at mile 3.3. Turn left on the spur trail and
look for Marys Rock at mile 3.4.

The panorama from the huge outcrop ranges far and wide. Choose your viewing spot. To the north there are easy views of many Blue Ridge peaks. The town of Luray and the Shenandoah Valley are visible to the west. Skilled climbers can walk to the highest rock and see in every direction. Decide for yourself if Marys Rock has the best view in the park. Just be careful doing it.

> **DIRECTIONS:** From Thornton Gap, take Skyline Drive south for 4.9 miles to the Jewell Hollow Overlook at milepost 36.4. Go to the far end of the overlook to the rock-walled parking area and look for the sign that says "Appalachian Trail 50 ft." Start your hike here.

Robertson Mountain

SCENERY: ☆ ☆ ☆ ☆ ☆
DIFFICULTY: ☆ ☆
TRAIL CONDITION: ☆ ☆ ☆ ☆
SOLITUDE: ☆ ☆ ☆
CHILDREN: ☆ ☆ ☆
DISTANCE: *6.2 miles round-trip*
HIKING TIME: *4:00 round-trip*
OUTSTANDING FEATURES: *great views, big trees*

ROBERTSON MOUNTAIN IS ONE OF THE PARK'S *best, but least visited, destinations. Reaching the rocky summit is neither difficult nor time-consuming, but most people pass it by to climb nearby Old Rag, one of the park's most crowded destinations. To get there, leave Skyline Drive and walk a portion of the Limberlost Trail, passing through a shady hemlock forest. A little footwork brings you to the outcrops of Robertson Mountain. There, various rocky points avail sweeping views in three directions. The crowds thin out just a short distance from Skyline Drive.*

🚶 To begin, take the gravelly Limberlost Trail from the parking area and enter a hemlock forest that Skyland Resort founder George Pollock helped protect nearly a century ago. Pass a horse path and Whiteoak Canyon Trail, to intersect the Old Rag Fire Road at 0.4 miles. Turn left onto the road where a sign reads, "Horse path, Skyland, Big Meadows." The fire road drops down, crossing Whiteoak Run. As you climb out of the drainage, stay left and look for big hemlocks beside the trail.

Stay on the fire road past two more bridle paths and a ranger station at mile 1. Continue down the

ROBERTSON MOUNTAIN

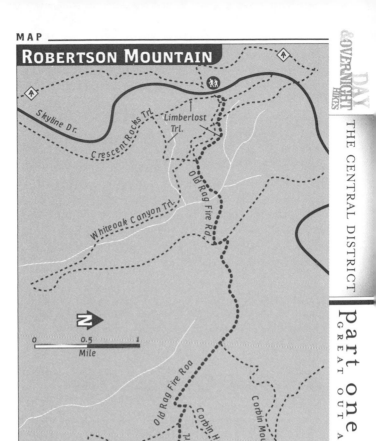

Skyline Dr.

Crescent Rocks Trl.

Limberlost Trl.

Old Rag Fire Rd.

Whiteoak Canyon Trl.

Old Rag Fire Roa

Corbin Hollow Trl.

Corbin Mountain Trl.

Robertson Mtn. Trl.

Robertson
Mtn.
3296

0   0.5   1
Mile

ELEVATION PROFILE

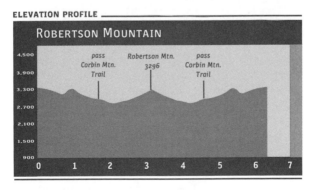

ROBERTSON MOUNTAIN

| | pass
Corbin Mtn.
Trail | Robertson Mtn.
3296 | pass
Corbin Mtn.
Trail |

side of Thorofare Mountain, passing huge oak trees
scattered amid the woods. The trail turns sharply to
the left and approaches the Corbin Mountain Trail
at mile 1.7. Keep descending gently on Old Rag past
more big trees.

Pass Corbin Hollow Trail at mile 2.2. Begin looking for the Robertson Mountain Trail just ahead where you will turn left. The footpath enters a laurel thicket, then turns back right.

The real climbing doesn't start for another quarter mile, where the path begins to switchback among rocks and trees. At mile 3.1, the trail passes the summit on your right. Look on your right for a spur trail leading to various outcrops. The depths of Whiteoak Canyon are below. Look for the cleared overlooks along Skyline Drive and the Blue Ridge. The hump of Hawksbill Mountain looms tall to the southwest. Views to the north are a little harder to find, but scout around. Take your time and take it all in; it's great being on top of this mountain.

> **DIRECTIONS:** From Thornton Gap, take Skyline Drive south for 12.5 miles to the Limberlost Trail parking area at milepost 43. The parking area is just a short distance to the left of Skyline Drive.

Whiteoak Canyon Falls

SCENERY: ✪ ✪ ✪ ✪ ✪
DIFFICULTY: ✪ ✪ ✪
TRAIL CONDITION: ✪ ✪ ✪
SOLITUDE: ✪
CHILDREN: ✪ ✪ ✪
DISTANCE: *5.6 miles round-trip*
HIKING TIME: *4:15 round-trip*
OUTSTANDING FEATURES: *Canyon views, six waterfalls*

IT'S HARD TO KEEP TRACK OF ALL THE FALLS *at Whiteoak Canyon. There are six sequentially numbered falls, starting from the Blue Ridge and ending down at the base of the canyon. Whether or not you correctly number the falls, take this classic Shenandoah hike, for there are not only falls but also canyon views and everywhere-you-look beauty.*

Leave from the rear of the parking area in Whiteoak Canyon and cross Cedar Run. When you reach the Cedar Run Trail junction at mile 0.2, veer right and soon cross Whiteoak Run. The trail gently follows the eastern side of the creek. You will pass a junction with the Cedar Run–Whiteoak Canyon Link Trail at 0.8 miles.

Here, many sycamore trees, which can be identified by their bark, line the stream. The lower trunks

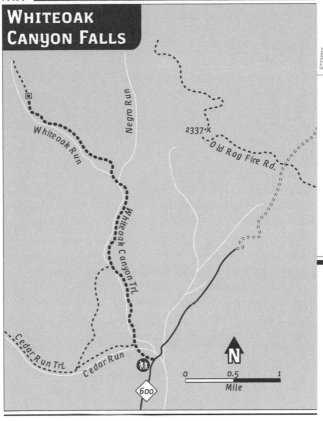

ELEVATION PROFILE

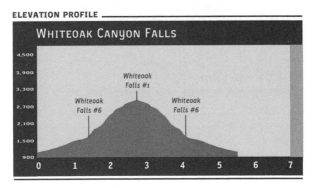

of sycamore trees have a tan bark; farther up the tree it looks as if the bark has peeled off, leaving a seemingly unhealthy but natural look. Tree spotters remember the adage "sycamores look sick."

Stay on the east bank of Whiteoak Run, entering a rock garden. On a moderate grade, pass Negro Run, which has a falls of its own, on your right. Just beyond this crossing close in on Whiteoak Falls (no. 6) at mile 1.5. A short trail leads left to the steep falls.

The main trail switchbacks, meandering far away from the stream. At mile 1.8, climb sharply along the base of a bluff. Soon, come to a lone cedar tree that mans an overlook into the canyon. Catch glimpses of the crashing falls below, and continue switchbacking up the canyon and below other cliffs. This is where the numbered falls get confusing. But enjoy the views and leave the counting to others.

The trail returns to Whiteoak Run and then to the base of another falls at mile 2.5. Pass an over-hanging boulder on your right. Keep climbing on rock steps. In some places, a combination of rock and concrete makes the pathway more hiker friendly.

A side trail at a concrete marker leads left to the base of Whiteoak Falls (no. 1) at mile 2.7. The main trail switchbacks to the right and comes to a rock observation point for Whiteoak Falls (no. 1). This is the second highest falls in the park at 86 feet. Rest and enjoy these falls and the good view into the canyon below. On your return trip try to count the falls. After all, Whiteoak Run has more falls per mile than any other stream in the park.

DIRECTIONS: From the town of Madison, drive north on VA 231 for 5 miles to VA 670. Turn left on VA 670 and follow it for 5 miles to VA 643. Turn right on VA 643 and follow it for less than a mile to VA 600. Turn left on VA 600 and follow it for 3.7 miles to Berry Hollow. The trailhead is in the back of the far parking area, which will be on your left.

Cedar Run Falls

SCENERY: ✿ ✿ ✿ ✿ ✿
DIFFICULTY: ✿ ✿ ✿
TRAIL CONDITION: ✿ ✿ ✿
SOLITUDE: ✿ ✿
CHILDREN: ✿ ✿ ✿
DISTANCE: *3.4 miles round-trip*
HIKING TIME: *3:15 round-trip*
OUTSTANDING FEATURES: *rugged gorge, falls*

THIS HIKE LEADS YOU INTO UPPER *Cedar Run Canyon. The trail down to the falls is steep as it passes innumerable cascades spilling down the narrow gorge. This place is wild and deserving of national park protection. Your trip to the falls will be slow, because you will need to watch your footing and often stop to admire the scenery.*

CEDAR RUN FALLS

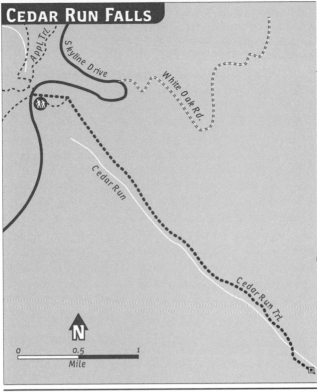

ELEVATION PROFILE

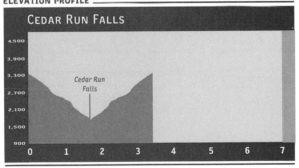

CEDAR RUN FALLS

Cedar Run
Falls

 Leave the parking area and grassy Hawksbill Gap behind to enter the woods on the Cedar Run Trail. Immediately coming to a trail junction, bear left. Hike a short distance and bear right at a second junction toward the "No Horses" sign. The trail grade drops sharply in a thick forest alongside the upper reaches of Cedar Run, as the white noise of cold mountain water serenades hikers all the way to the falls.

Large oaks are scattered along the rocky trail. A side branch crosses the trail at 0.6 miles, forming a cascade of its own. Soon, you'll walk alongside the fast-moving run. Step onto the wide rock, facing a cascade, to your right. Cedar Run descends 20 feet in a fan pattern then crashes onto the rock on which you are standing.

Beyond this cascade the trail drops steeply alongside a stair-step cascade to your right and a rocky bluff to your left. The trail comes back to Cedar Run near a large fallen oak that spans the river. Below this, Cedar Run circumvents an island, and the trail winds below a second cliff to a ford at mile 1.5. This is usually a rock hop; however, it can be a wet crossing at high water.

Across the stream the trail climbs briefly, passing a feeder stream trickling in from your right. The Cedar Run Trail descends a set of stone steps to the base of Cedar Run Falls at mile 1.7. The water spills down a slick rock face and lands in a plunge pool, then it drops even more. Many large boulders make good relaxing and observation points. You can go a bit farther downstream to enjoy these falls from a different perspective. The hike back is ambitious (i.e., very steep), so pace yourself.

DIRECTIONS: From Thornton Gap, take Skyline Drive south for 14.1 miles to Hawksbill Gap at milepost 45.6. The Cedar Run trail starts behind the gravel parking area located to the left of Skyline Drive.

Hawksbill Summit

SCENERY: ✰ ✰ ✰ ✰ ✰
DIFFICULTY: ✰
TRAIL CONDITION: ✰ ✰ ✰ ✰
SOLITUDE: ✰
CHILDREN: ✰ ✰ ✰ ✰ ✰
DISTANCE: 2.2 miles round-trip
HIKING TIME: 1:30 round-trip
OUTSTANDING FEATURES: highest viewpoint in the entire park

THIS IS AN EASY, FAVORITE HIKE THAT starts at a high elevation and gets to the top of things in Shenandoah. Along the way you'll enter a "sky island" of Canadian-type forest. Outcrops below the summit are just warm-ups for the nearly 360-degree view from the summit of Hawksbill.

🏃 Leave from the back of the Upper Hawksbill parking area onto the wide and gravelly Hawksbill Mountain Trail. The trail makes a quick jump and

HAWKSBILL SUMMIT

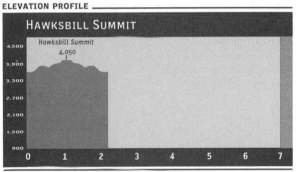

ELEVATION PROFILE

continues at a moderate grade. The small logs or "waterbars" across the trailbed help prevent erosion during prolonged rains and thunderstorms that sometimes wrack the Blue Ridge.

At this elevation the growing season is short; the trees don't begin to foliate until late May. Late September finds leaves turning as trees prepare for a cold season that's longer than in the adjoining valleys.

At 0.4 miles the trail levels and actually descends to reach the Hawksbill Mountain Fire Road at 0.6 miles. Turn right and head up the gullied fire road through an area damaged by gypsy moths. The road climbs steeply while veering to the right. Turn left up a narrow footpath and immediately bear right. This is the Salamander Trail. Watch for a double blue blaze on a tree to your left at 0.9 miles.

Here you will begin to see balsam fir and red spruce, components of the Canadian-type (or Boreal) forest that covered much of Shenandoah thousands of years ago. As the climate warmed and the ancient glaciers receded, these trees clung to the highest peaks of the Appalachians, forming "sky islands" of these Canadian plant communities.

The Salamander Trail travels just a short distance to a trail junction. Bear right and swing around by some rock outcrops. Take in some inspiring views to the west. Soon, you'll come to the day-use shelter, Byrds Nest No. 2.

Ascend briefly and step up onto the Hawksbill (4,050 feet). Though the exposed rocks provide good overlooks, the man-made observation platform may help you orient yourself. Metal plates showing the cardinal points are laid into the rock walls of the platform. And what views you'll find: Old Rag, Stony Man, Crescent Rock, and Nakedtop, as well as towns and hollows in the Shenandoah Valley. It's a good feeling—being on top of the Blue Ridge.

DIRECTIONS: From Thornton Gap, take Skyline Drive south for 15.2 miles to Upper Hawksbill parking area at milepost 46.7. The Hawksbill Mountain Trail starts at the back of the parking area.

Bear Church Rock

> SCENERY: ✿ ✿ ✿ ✿ ✿
> DIFFICULTY: ✿ ✿
> TRAIL CONDITION: ✿ ✿ ✿ ✿ ✿
> SOLITUDE: ✿ ✿ ✿ ✿ ✿
> CHILDREN: ✿ ✿
> DISTANCE: *9 miles round-trip*
> HIKING TIME: *3:30 round-trip*
> OUTSTANDING FEATURES: *great views, isolated ridge hiking*

THIS HIGH-COUNTRY HIKE TRAVERSES *the ridge of Jones Mountain to an incredible view from Bear Church Rock. The hiking along Jones Mountain is some of Shenandoah's finest. It's never steep for long and is level much of the way. The entire hike is on foot trails that meander through varied and beautiful forests. This is a great way to spend a day in Shenandoah. Make sure you carry water.*

🚶 To begin, head north on the Appalachian Trail from Bootens Gap. The AT moderately ascends

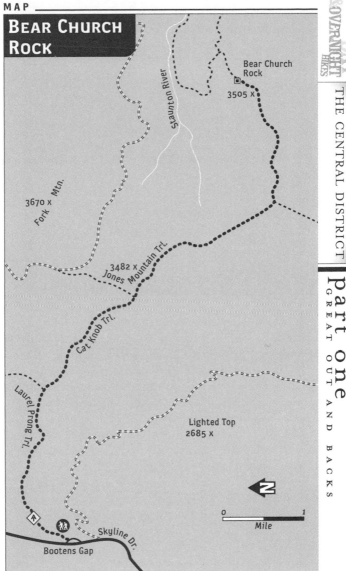

the southwest side of Hazeltop, coming to a trail junction at 0.4 miles. Turn right on Laurel Prong Trail, descending past several springs on a boulder-laden slope. Just before arriving at the breezy Laurel Gap and another trail junction at mile 1.4, the trail drops sharply .

Continue forward on Cat Knob Trail. The trail winds uphill, twisting and turning among large gray boulders. Leave the National Park and enter a slice of the Rapidan Wildlife Management Area at mile

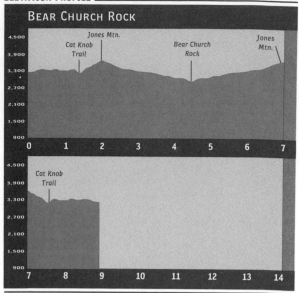

BEAR CHURCH ROCK

1.8. The trail makes one last jump and a slight descent before intersecting the Jones Mountain Trail at mile 2.1. Turn right on the Jones Mountain Trail.

This ridge-running path makes for pleasant walking among windswept oaks. The fern and grass understory, mingled with mountain laurel, makes the path even more appealing. The little-used trail descends, making an unexpected right turn at mile 2.6. Reach a gap in a broken forest, where the brush may crowd the path in late summer. Reenter Shenandoah National Park at mile 2.9 in an oak woodland. Begin an extensive stretch that descends slightly. The scenery is among the park's finest.

In a grassy gap at mile 3.5, the trail turns left and heads down, descending east toward Bear Church Rock and away from Bluff Mountain. Look for an outcrop on your left that has views of Fork Mountain. Begin a downward roller-coaster ride through Jones Mountain among large granite out-crops in the woods. Watch your footing.

At mile 4.4 the trail zigzags very steeply down the point of the ridge through brush and laurel. In 0.1 mile, watch for a side trail to the left, which emerges onto the granite slab of Bear Church Rock, a natural viewing platform. What a perch! Some claim the view is a near-religious experience, at least for bruins. Fork Mountain, Doubletop Mountain, and the crest of the Blue Ridge stand out. Below you is the

Staunton River. Both bears and humans will be moved on Bear Church Rock.

> **DIRECTIONS:** From Swift Run Gap, head north on Skyline Drive for 10.4 miles to the Bootens Gap parking area (mile 55.3). The small parking area is on your right. The Appalachian Trail skirts the back of the parking area.

South River Cemetery
via Pocosin Trail

SCENERY: ☆ ☆ ☆
TRAIL CONDITION: ☆ ☆ ☆
CHILDREN: ☆ ☆ ☆
DIFFICULTY: ☆ ☆
SOLITUDE: ☆ ☆ ☆
DISTANCE: *5 miles round-trip*
HIKING TIME: *3:30 round-trip*
OUTSTANDING FEATURES: *Pocosin Mission, homesites, big tree, pioneer cemetery*

THIS IS AN HISTORICAL HIKE, *taking you through numerous old homesteads. Drop from the high country to a gap and the Pocosin Mission, where a brave Episcopalian minister tried to save the souls of the surrounding mountaineers. Then take the seldom-used Pocosin Trail past homesites and a huge tulip tree to reach the South River Cemetery, a resting place being reclaimed by nature. On your return trip you can look for less obvious signs of a pre-park past.*

🐾 Leave the parking area on the nearly level grade of the Pocosin Fire Road to cross the Appalachian Trail at mile 0.1. At 0.2 miles, in a clearing, is the Pocosin Cabin, built in 1937 by the Civilian Conservation Corps. The Potomac Appalachian Trail Club rents this cabin; call (703) 242-0693 to make a reservation or visit www.patc.net/activities/cabins/ for more information. The fire road continues dropping and the wide-open double track centered by grass makes for easy walking. Before you know it, reach a junction at 1 mile. Through the trees to your right are the remains of the Pocosin Mission. Follow the footpath to the steps of the old church, built in 1904. Look at the walls made of native stone. Another nearby building is barely standing. Parts of the structure were built with hand-hewn logs. Boards, nails, and even tarpaper were later additions. Another building foundation has a fallen stone chimney, nearly intact,

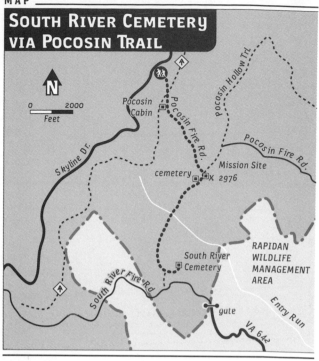

SOUTH RIVER CEMETERY VIA POCOSIN TRAIL

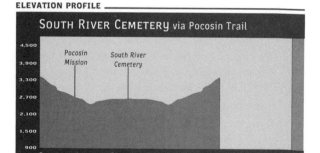

ELEVATION PROFILE

SOUTH RIVER CEMETERY via Pocosin Trail

behind it. Look for the cemetery where a few graves are marked with simple stones.

Heading roughly south, leave the Pocosin Mission on the Pocosin Trail. The concrete trail post states, "South River Fire Road, 1.5." Descend along a streamlet, crossing the small watercourse at 1.2 miles. Cruise along a mountainside to reach Entry Run, which the aforementioned streamlet meets far below the trail. Entry Run is wide, shallow, and easily walked across. Notice chunks of asphalt on the trail, indicating this little-used footpath was once a road. Look also for small pieces of glass on the trail below

Entry Run. A sharp eye will also spot metal relics in the adjacent woods, indicating a former homesite. The small stream running under the trail by culvert was the homesteaders likely water source. On your return trip look for parts of an old jalopy.

At 2.1 miles, a massive tulip tree stands next to the trail. This behemoth can't be missed. What changes the tree has seen over time! Climb away from the giant, circling uphill around a feeder branch of Entry Run. Reach a gap grown over in locust trees, then come to a trail junction at mile 2.4. The access path to South River Cemetery is dead ahead, while the Pocosin Trail leaves right to shortly meet South River Fire Road. Keep forward for 0.1 mile on the narrow access path to reach South River Cemetery. A dilapidated wood and wire fence circles the inter-ment area. Pass though the tilting gate. A large head-stone made of quartz boulders stands out. Others range from clearly marked recent stones to flat field-stones or mere depressions in the ground. The cemetery is losing the battle against nature and is being reclaimed. Cherry trees grow overhead inside the fence and the forest outside the fence is crowding in. The evolving forest has no regard for human bur-ial sites. Unless you have a shovel, a pine box, and a yearning for a long nap, return the way you came.

DIRECTIONS: From Swift Run Gap, drive north on Skyline Drive for 6 miles to mile 59.5. Look on your right for a road with a sign that states, "Do Not Block Fire Road." Turn on this road and park in one of the gravel spots. The Pocosin Fire Road starts here.

Lost Cliffs

SCENERY: ✿ ✿ ✿ ✿ ✿
TRAIL CONDITION: ✿ ✿ ✿
CHILDREN: ✿
DIFFICULTY: ✿ ✿ ✿
SOLITUDE: ✿ ✿ ✿ ✿ ✿
DISTANCE: *2.4 miles round-trip*
HIKING TIME: *2:30 round-trip*
OUTSTANDING FEATURES: *views from Lost Cliffs, solitude, small cascade*

MAYBE THESE CLIFFS SHOULD BE NAMED *the "Forgotten Cliffs."
It seems no one comes here, though a fantastic view from atop the
cliffs allows hikers to easily orient themselves, and not feel "lost."*

LOST CLIFFS

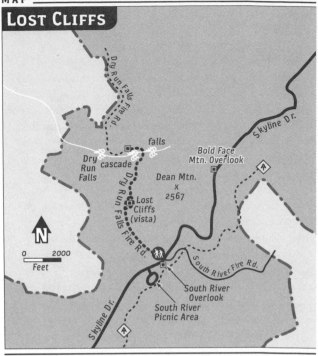

The hike follows Dry Run Falls Fire Road away from Skyline Drive to pass the cliffs. A not-too-difficult, 75-yard, uphill scramble is necessary to reach the clifftops and the views, but is not recommended for families with younger children. Beyond the cliffs, this hike leads down to Dry Run, a forgotten stream with a small trailside cascade. The actual Dry Run Falls can be accessed with some rough bushwhacking and is recommended only for the intrepid explorer. The Trail Condition and Difficulty rating above may be confusing, as the Dry Run Falls Fire Road is open and well maintained with a moderate grade, but the manway for the short scramble is unmaintained. The rating considers both situations.

Cross Skyline Drive from the parking area and head northwest on the Dry Run Falls Fire Road. Stately oaks flank the level road at its entrance. Pass around a yellow chain gate and join the yellow-blazed path. Soon begin a steady descent among tall hardwoods. Look downhill to your left for an abandoned settler road running alongside Dry Run Falls Fire Road.

At 0.7 miles, the Lost Cliffs come into view. The massive, tilted outcrop lifts skyward from the mountainside to your right. Big boulders and smaller rocks, eroded from the cliffs, litter the woods below the outcrop. Keep downhill, reaching the lower end of the cliffs. Look right for a rough manway heading

ELEVATION PROFILE

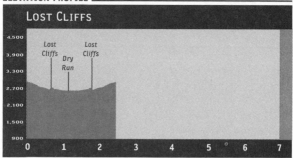

directly uphill from the fire road. Follow this faint path up through the woods then veer right onto the cliff face. Barley discernible paths run along the edge of the cliffs. The farther you go along the cliffs, the more you rise and the more views open until the whole of the Shenandoah Valley, Massanutten Mountain, and other lands to the west expand before your eyes. Savor this view and take your time. It is likely that no one will interrupt this natural moment. To leave the Lost Cliffs and return to the fire road, keep along the cliff's edge until the steepness forces you into the woods behind the cliffs and circle back down to the fire road. Be very careful on the cliffs.

Continue down the fire road, moving beyond the cliffs, and pass a rocked-in spring to the right of the fire road at 1 mile. The spring's outflow crosses the trail. Curve into the Dry Run watershed, reaching Dry Run at mile 1.2. A sign posting park fishing regulations is at the creek. Rock hop Dry Run and head downstream just a short distance. To your left is a small cascade tumbling over boulders. For most of us, this fall, which can turn nearly dry in late summer and fall, will have to suffice as the hike's destination. Reaching Dry Run Falls necessitates rough bushwhacking through fallen trees, especially dying hemlock trees under attack from the hemlock woolly adelgid, a bug that defoliates the hemlocks. Yet another waterfall is upstream of the Dry Run Fall Fire Road crossing, but it, too, is tough to reach.

DIRECTIONS: From Swift Run Gap, drive north on Skyline Drive for 2.8 miles, parking at the South River Overlook, just beyond the right turn into South River Picnic Area. Dry Run Falls Fire Road starts just uproad on the western side of Skyline Drive, opposite the side of the parking area. Do not take the South River Fire Road, which starts just uproad and on the same side as the parking area.

South River Falls

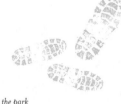

SCENERY: ✿ ✿ ✿ ✿
DIFFICULTY: ✿ ✿
TRAIL CONDITION: ✿ ✿ ✿ ✿ ✿
SOLITUDE: ✿
CHILDREN: ✿ ✿ ✿ ✿
DISTANCE: *3.8 miles round-trip*
HIKING TIME: *2:30 round-trip*
OUTSTANDING FEATURES: *third highest falls in the park*

GRAVITY PLAYS A BIG ROLE IN THIS HIKE. *Make an easy descent and see South River Falls drop 80 feet over a rock face. Go farther and enjoy the view from the base of the falls. You'll have to fight the earth's tug on your climb out of the South River watershed, back to the former mountaintop pastureland; but the falls are worth the climb.*

🚶 Leave from the rear of the South River Picnic Area on a wide dirt footpath (South River Falls Trail) and cross the Appalachian Trail at 0.1 mile. Continue down to a switchback at 0.4 miles. Twist and turn three more times before coming to the South River, which is just a small creek at this point. Cross a side branch and enjoy the lush streamside environment.

Look for yellow birch; its pale, yellow-gray, peeling bark has vertical lines running through it. This tree likes moist, cool environments. There are many hemlocks as well, though most are dying or dead, thanks to the invasive woolly adelgid.

Come to a second tributary at mile 0.9. Ahead and to your right is the top of the falls, but keep going—there's a better and safer viewpoint a short distance past the granite wall to your left. Walk out on the outcrop to your right and see South River Falls. There is so much more light here than in the dark streamside environment. South River Falls is spotlighted as well.

Water plunges down a rock face into a small pool then cascades into a second pool. The water is slowly, unceasingly cutting into the rock face. Saddleback Mountain is off to your left. For a different perspective continue down the trail, passing a trail junction. Veer right and descend to river level again. Head upriver on a foot trail and come to the base of the falls at mile 1.9. Looking up, you can see how the watercourse splits nearly in two before resuming a calmer path to the sea.

MAP

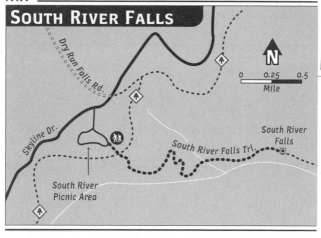

SOUTH RIVER FALLS

Dry Run Falls Rd.

N

0   0.25   0.5
Mile

Skyline Dr.

South River Falls Trl.

South River Falls

South River Picnic Area

ELEVATION PROFILE

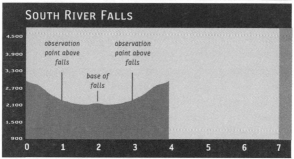

SOUTH RIVER FALLS

4,500
3,900
3,300
2,700
2,100
1,500
900

observation point above falls

observation point above falls

base of falls

0   1   2   3   4   5   6   7

DIRECTIONS: From Swift Run Gap, drive north on Skyline Drive for 2.7 miles to South River Picnic Area (mile 63), which will be on your right. Head to the back of the picnic area on the one-way loop road. The trailhead will be on your right.

Hightop Peak

SCENERY: ✿ ✿ ✿ ✿ ✿
DIFFICULTY: ✿ ✿
TRAIL CONDITION: ✿ ✿ ✿ ✿
SOLITUDE: ✿ ✿ ✿
CHILDREN: ✿ ✿ ✿ ✿ ✿
DISTANCE: *3.4 miles round-trip*
HIKING TIME: *2:30 round-trip*
OUTSTANDING FEATURES: *mountain vistas from the highest peak in the South District*

THIS IS ONE PEAK MOST EVERYONE can bag. Just at the point where novice hikers get tired of climbing, the path tops out and offers a very rewarding view. Get a taste of the Appalachian Trail (AT) while climbing one of the park's higher mountains.

🚶 Start this hike by crossing Skyline Drive from the Hightop Mountain parking area and heading south on the AT. Walk through a grassy area on a moderate uphill grade, passing two boulders that act as sentinels for the mountaintop. Ahead, more gray boulders line the path, which becomes rocky as it climbs. You will cross an older and steeper trail at 0.5 miles. A level section offers a brief reprieve before the AT starts switchbacking up the mountain at a steeper grade.

At mile 1.1 the trail again levels. The larger oak and tulip trees at this elevation take on a gnarled appearance; the weather can be rough up here and the trees show it. But nature has a gentler side on Hightop, too, that is evident by the trilliums and other wildflowers that bloom in spring—late May and early June up here.

The trail swings around the right side of Hightop, soon passing two outcrops that offer first-rate vistas. The first outcrop reveals Massanutten Peak straight ahead. To your right is the town of Elkton and, of course, the Shenandoah Valley. The cluster of houses just below is Sandy Bottom.

The next outcrop, also to the right of the trail, is even more spectacular. Plainly visible is the rock face of Rocky Mount. The bulk of Shenandoah's mountains extend in the distance, wave upon wave. The mass of mountain to your left is Flattop Mountain, and Skyline Drive is just below you.

Continue just a short distance farther until you come to a trace of an old trail leading left. Get to the

HIGHTOP PEAK

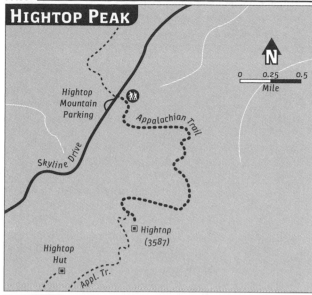

ELEVATION PROFILE

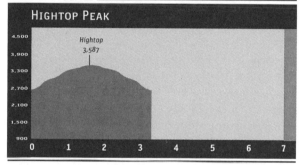

top of Hightop (3,587 feet) at mile 1.7. There are
few views here since the fire tower was dismantled,
but it makes a good lunch spot if the winds are high
on the outcrops. Congratulations, you've gained
nearly 1,000 feet of altitude in less than 2 miles.

DIRECTIONS: From Swift Run Gap drive south on Skyline
Drive for 1.2 miles to Hightop Mountain parking area (mile
66.7), which will be on your right.

Furnace Mountain *via Blackrock*

ONCE YOU FINISH ENJOYING THE *outstanding views from Blackrock Summit with other hikers, leave the crowds behind to enter one of the park's more remote areas, Furnace Mountain. Be careful; the trail is rocky, so take your time and enjoy the solitude.*

🚶 Leave the rear of the Blackrock Summit parking area on the wide roadbed of the Trayfoot Mountain Trail. Begin climbing and intersect the narrower Appalachian Trail (AT) at 0.1 mile. Head south on the level-running AT to intersect the Blackrock Spur Trail at 0.4 miles, passing through a rock jumble with fine views into Dundo Hollow to your right. Turn right onto the Blackrock Spur Trail and descend, passing between some very large boulders. Trayfoot Mountain is close and to your left. Furnace Mountain is beyond Trayfoot Mountain and to your right. Intersect the Trayfoot Mountain Trail at 0.5 miles.

Turn right on the Trayfoot Mountain Trail and descend to a gap then begin climbing a grassy ridge with many dead trees, victims of the gypsy moth. The moths, which defoliate trees, were introduced to the northeastern United States from Europe in 1869. Unfortunately they reached Shenandoah in 1983.

At mile 1.6 you'll come to your fourth trail junction. Leave the Trayfoot Mountain Trail and turn right onto the Furnace Mountain Trail. Drop down the northern flank of Trayfoot Mountain and pass through a talus slope, where the loose rock makes bad footing. The trail loses elevation steadily, making two sharp turns—first to the left, then to the right—arriving at a gap at mile 2.4. The ridge narrows here as you cross an open forest of pine and mountain laurel.

Come to a spur trail near the Furnace Mountain summit at mile 3.2. Turn right onto the spur trail

FURNACE MOUNTAIN VIA BLACKROCK

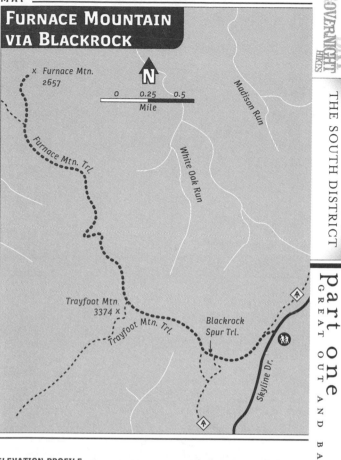

Furnace Mtn. 2657

Furnace Mtn. Trl.

Madison Run

White Oak Run

N

0   0.25   0.5
Mile

Trayfoot Mtn. 3374

Trayfoot Mtn. Trl.

Blackrock Spur Trl.

Skyline Dr.

ELEVATION PROFILE

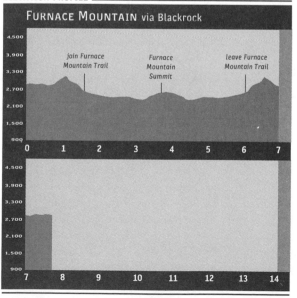

FURNACE MOUNTAIN via Blackrock

join Furnace Mountain Trail

Furnace Mountain Summit

leave Furnace Mountain Trail

and begin climbing. As you climb, wide views of the Shenandoah Valley open to your left. Descend slightly on the north side of Furnace Mountain to reach a rock outcrop overlooking the lower canyon of Madison Run in Dundo Hollow. Directly across the canyon is Austin Mountain. To your right is the main crest of the Blue Ridge. Relax and enjoy the view; you'll most likely have it all to yourself.

DIRECTIONS: From Rockfish Gap entrance station, head north on Skyline Drive for 19.9 miles to Blackrock Summit parking area (mile 84.8) on your left.

Big Branch Falls
via Moormans River

SCENERY: ☆ ☆ ☆ ☆
DIFFICULTY: ☆ ☆
TRAIL CONDITION: ☆ ☆ ☆
SOLITUDE: ☆ ☆ ☆ ☆ ☆
CHILDREN: ☆ ☆ ☆
DISTANCE: *6.8 miles round-trip*
HIKING TIME: *4:15 round-trip*
OUTSTANDING FEATURES: *Big Branch Falls, flood-scoured gorge, solitude*

IF YOU WOULD LIKE TO SEE AN EXAMPLE *of the raw power of nature, take this hike. Big Branch Falls is a worthy destination, but it is the incredible power of the 1995 flood on the north fork of the Moormans River gorge that you will remember.*

🐾 Your hike leaves Blackrock Gap (2,330 feet) to descend moderately on the Moormans River Fire Road. At 0.1 mile, cross a small branch of the river that the trail begins to parallel. Pass an area containing many dead pine trees. The trees are victims of the Southern pine beetle, an indigenous insect that ravages pine forests in cycles. The rest of the slope is covered with mountain laurel.

At mile 1.1, come to a gate on the road. Leaving the park, the trail descends to a junction at mile 1.4. Turn right and cross the North Fork Moormans River on rocks. The trail follows the river downstream. At mile 1.6, turn right at another junction and pass a ramshackle hunters camp on your left. Look for the smooth gray trunks of the many beech trees that grow in the area. Their nuts are a favored wildlife food source.

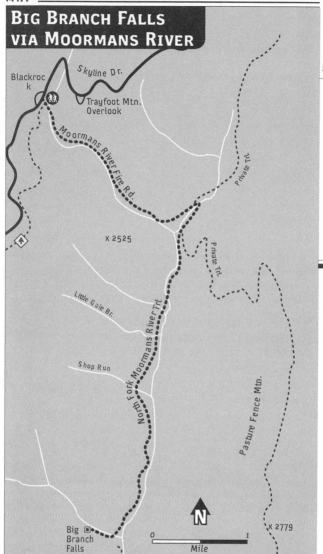

BIG BRANCH FALLS VIA MOORMANS RIVER

Skyline Dr.

Blackrock

Trayfoot Mtn. Overlook

Moormans River Fire Rd.

Private Trl.

X 2525

Private Trl.

Little Gale Br.

North Fork Moormans River Trl.

Shop Run

Pasture Fence Mtn.

Big Branch Falls

N

0   1
Mile

X 2779

ELEVATION PROFILE

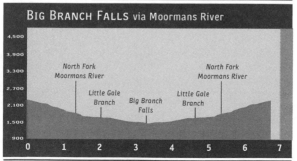

BIG BRANCH FALLS via Moormans River

4,500

3,900

3,300   North Fork   North Fork
        Moormans River   Moormans River

2,700
        Little Gale   Little Gale
2,100   Branch   Big Branch   Branch
                    Falls
1,500

900
    0   1   2   3   4   5   6   7

Make another easy rock hop across the river at mile 1.8. You will stay on the western bank for the remainder of the hike. Reenter the park at the crossing of Little Gale Branch. After the road takes on a more overgrown appearance, you'll soon see the first evidence of the 1995 flood—a massive mudslide that thundered down from your right, sweeping away trees and vegetation. Leave the mudslide area and gently ascend. To your left are views of Pasture Fence Mountain.

Cross Shop Run at mile 2.5 and make a fair descent into a second washed out area that is much more rocky than the first. This is just the precursor for the biggest slide, which extends to both sides of the river. The flood scoured the valley here; there is nothing but rock, soil, and piles of downed trees. Changes in nature often occur imperceptibly, but here the sudden, violent, and lasting power of the elements was unleashed on the north fork of Moormans River.

Come to Big Branch at mile 3.3. Though a 0.1-mile side trail leads right to the falls on the far side of Big Branch, thanks to the flood, you can see Big Branch Falls from the main trail. This canyon was gouged out too, exposing the rocky bed of the creek. The low-volume falls drop 30 feet into a pool and another cascade slides into a second pool. On your return trip imagine, if you can, this creek and the Moormans River during the violent flood of 1995.

> DIRECTIONS: From the Rockfish Gap entrance station take Skyline Drive north for 17.2 miles to Blackrock Gap parking area at milepost 87.4, which will be on your left.

Chimney Rock

SCENERY: ✿ ✿ ✿ ✿ ✿
DIFFICULTY: ✿ ✿
TRAIL CONDITION: ✿ ✿ ✿ ✿
SOLITUDE: ✿ ✿
CHILDREN: ✿ ✿ ✿ ✿
DISTANCE: *3.4 miles round-trip*
HIKING TIME: *2:15 round-trip*
OUTSTANDING FEATURES: *views from Chimney Rock*

BE CAREFUL WHEN YOU GET TO CHIMNEY ROCK. *A deep crevasse separates the actual Chimney Rock and the rock you can reach safely. At one time a short bridge spanned this crevasse, but only the*

MAP

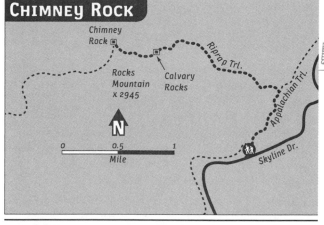

ELEVATION PROFILE

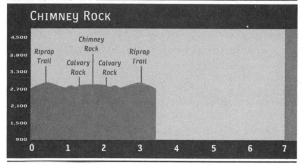

metal anchors remain. Note that in October 1998 and May 1999, two major wildland fires swept through this area. The effects are evident along portions of the Riprap Trail and Appalachian Trail (AT).

The hike starts on the Riprap Trail. Leave the Riprap parking area and walk a grand total of 100 feet before intersecting the Appalachian Trail. Turn right on the AT and climb north through a pine and oak forest with a thick understory of azaleas and mountain laurel. These shrubs display their pink blooms in May and June. Intersect the continuation of the Riprap Trail at 0.4 miles.

Turn left on the Riprap Trail. It makes a sharp switchback to the right at 0.5 miles then begins to descend, passing through a chestnut oak forest. A chestnut oak has thick leaves with wavy, rounded lobes on both sides of the leaf. Its acorns have been a primary food source for park animals since the demise of the chestnut tree in the early 1900s. Notice also a primary understory tree of the chestnut oak forest, the striped maple. It is distinguished by its vertically striped bark and large goose foot-shaped leaves.

The Riprap Trail comes to a gap at mile 1 and begins to climb, entering a rock field. The trail quickly veers to the right and then to the left, achieving the crest of the ridge. Immediately to your right is an outcrop with fine views into Paine Run below. An old gnarled pine tree by the trail offers substantial shade for the hot hiker.

Continue heading west on the narrow ridge past a series of boulders. This is all part of Rocks Mountain. The Calvary Rocks are reached at 1.4 miles. The forest has reclaimed this outcrop, which offered views in days gone by. Pass another boulder field and come to the side trail leading to Chimney Rock at mile 1.7. Turn right on the side trail and, a few steps later, emerge on the outcrop.

Carefully step out. Look below into the crevasse. Now look out from left to right. First you'll see the patchwork quilt of land that is the Shenandoah Valley and, beyond, the Alleghenies. Below you'll see Paine Run. The bulk in front of you is Trayfoot Mountain, which at 3,374 feet is the second highest peak in the South District. Finally, to your right is the Blue Ridge. There is plenty to see from here, even without a bridge to Chimney Rock.

DIRECTIONS: From Rockfish Gap entrance station, head north on Skyline Drive for 14.6 miles to Riprap parking area (mile 90) on your left.

Chimney Rock *via Riprap Hollow*

SCENERY: ✪ ✪ ✪ ✪ ✪
DIFFICULTY: ✪ ✪ ✪
TRAIL CONDITION: ✪ ✪ ✪
SOLITUDE: ✪ ✪
CHILDREN: ✪ ✪
DISTANCE: *6.8 miles round-trip*
HIKING TIME: *3:30 round-trip*
OUTSTANDING FEATURES: *canyon, swimming hole, views from Chimney Rock*

AS YOU MAKE YOUR WAY UP RIPRAP HOLLOW, *your environment will go through dramatic changes. Start out in a lush streamside forest, pass through a narrow canyon to a deep swimming hole, and emerge into a piney, rocky area. Then, ascend a vegetation-choked hollow to*

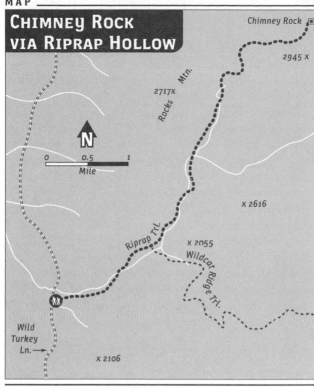

CHIMNEY ROCK VIA RIPRAP HOLLOW

Chimney Rock

2945 x

2717x

Rocks Mtn.

x 2616

Riprap Trl.

x 2055

Wildcat Ridge Trl.

Wild Turkey Ln. →

x 2106

N

0   0.5   1
Mile

ELEVATION PROFILE

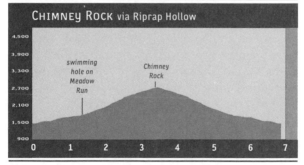

CHIMNEY ROCK via Riprap Hollow

4,500
3,900
3,300
2,700
2,100
1,500
900

swimming hole on Meadow Run

Chimney Rock

0   1   2   3   4   5   6   7

emerge onto the ridgetop with views from airy quartz outcrops. Bring your camera with you on this hike. In October 1998 and again in May 1999, two major wildland fires swept through this area. The effects are evident along portions of the Riprap and Wildcat Ridge Trails.

   👣 Leave the parking area on Riprap Trail, cross a small stream and reach the park boundary and a trail marker. Continue forward on a rocky roadbed that enters a pretty forest of pine and hardwoods. At 0.5 miles the nearly level trail crosses Meadow Run, the watercourse that flows through Riprap

Hollow. Look for a large white pine on trail-left that contrasts with the defoliated woodland up the canyon.

At 0.9 miles pass the Wildcat Ridge Trail junction, continuing forward. After passing a boulder field to your left, the canyon narrows, and the trail passes close to the stream. Here you may see Catawba rhododendron (rare in these parts) display its pink plumage around the first of June.

Cross Meadow Run at mile 1.4 and approach the swimming hole. Meadow Run makes a deep pool here, luring in hot and sweaty hikers. A set of rock steps leads to the pool. The trail crosses Meadow Run again and climbs briefly to a flat spot with a "No Camping" sign. Another sign points to the Riprap Trail, dead ahead. Do not take the trail to the right; it has been rerouted out of the canyon for safety.

Climb to an open area of rock and pine. Here you can look back down the hollow. Ahead the trail closes up again, entering a narrow section of the canyon. Notice the falls in the narrowest section of the canyon. Veer into the heavily wooded Cold Spring Hollow to the left at mile 1.8, where many birch and hemlock trees grow.

The trail climbs ever more abruptly, emerging onto Rocks Mountain at mile 2.8. Look for an outcrop with views into Paine Run Hollow. Continue east on the ridge, coming to a side trail at mile 3.4. Walk a few feet and you are at Chimney Rock, where the views open before you. Look below to Paine Run; beyond it lies the Shenandoah Valley. The massive mountain in front of you is Trayfoot Mountain. To the right of Trayfoot is the Blue Ridge.

DIRECTIONS: From the junction of US 250 and US 340 in Waynesboro (near Rockfish Gap), take US 340 north for 5.8 miles to VA 612. Turn right on VA 612 and follow it for 1.7 miles to Black Bear Lane. Turn left and follow Black Bear Lane a short distance to Wild Turkey Lane. Veer left on Wild Turkey Lane; you will reach the Riprap trailhead in 1.1 mile.

Turk Mountain

SCENERY: ✪ ✪ ✪ ✪ ✪
DIFFICULTY: ✪
TRAIL CONDITION: ✪ ✪ ✪
SOLITUDE: ✪ ✪ ✪
CHILDREN: ✪ ✪ ✪ ✪ ✪
DISTANCE: *2.2 miles round-trip*
HIKING TIME: *1:45 round-trip*
OUTSTANDING FEATURES: *great views from the summit of Turk Mountain*

TURK MOUNTAIN MAKES A GREAT INITIATION *hike for park visitors entering Shenandoah from the southern end. But no matter where you come from, you will not be disappointed by the outstanding views of this rocky mountain summit. The ample reward at trail's end outweighs the effort required to reach Shenandoah's most southwestern peak.*

🚶 Start your hike at Turk Gap. Cross Skyline Drive from the parking area and begin descending south on the Appalachian Trail, which immediately enters a stand of pines. Be sure to take the trail to the left once you cross the road. The trail to the right is the Turk Gap Trail. Soon you'll begin to climb and eventually arrive at a trail junction at 0.2 miles. Veer right onto the Turk Mountain Trail and descend to an unnamed gap at 0.5 miles.

The trail climbs the east slope of Turk Mountain amid an oak forest and soon enters a rock field. Continue through the rock field and come to a sharp right turn at mile 1. You can scramble onto the rocks to your left for views, but the rocks are unstable and the views are better atop the summit. The trail continues to the right, then goes between some large boulders just before attaining the crest of Turk Mountain.

At the crest, turn right to emerge onto an elevated rock outcrop and the summit of Turk Mountain (2,981 feet) at 1.1 mile. The views, especially to the west, are expansive, due to the talus slope extending far down the west flank of Turk Mountain. Beyond the talus slope is the Shenandoah Valley. On the far side of the valley are the Allegheny Mountains and the George Washington National Forest. Back to the east is Bucks Elbow Mountain with its radio towers. To the south is Calf Mountain, also with radio towers. To the north is Cool Spring Hollow and the undulating bulk of the park.

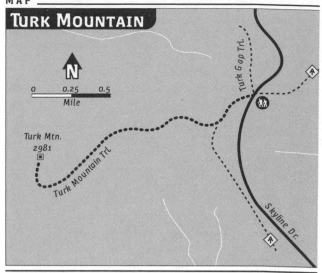

TURK MOUNTAIN

Turk Mtn.
2981

Turk Mountain Trl.

Turk Gap Trl.

Skyline Dr.

N

0   0.25   0.5
Mile

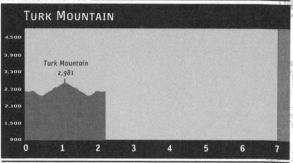

TURK MOUNTAIN

Turk Mountain
2,981

4,500
3,900
3,300
2,700
2,100
1,500
900

0   1   2   3   4   5   6   7

DIRECTIONS: From the Rockfish Gap entrance station take Skyline Drive north for 10.5 miles to Turk Gap parking area (mile 94.1), which will be on your right.

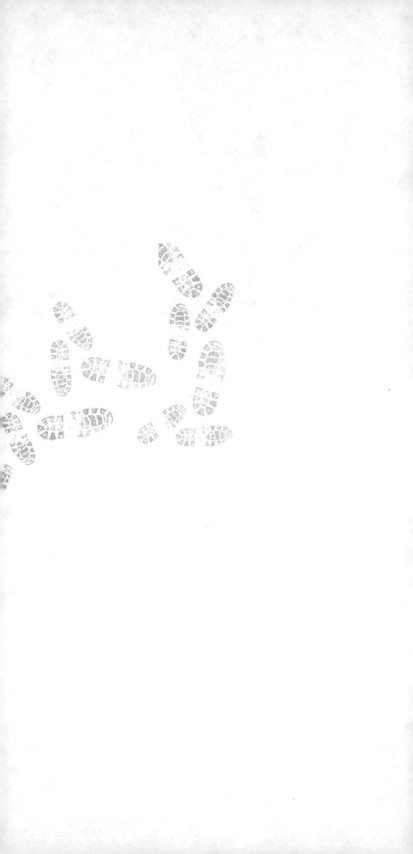

part two
GREAT DAY LOOPS

The return trip to the AT will get you huffing and puffing, while thinking of all the people that skipped this second view as is evidenced by the much less used trail tread.

Sugarloaf Loop

SCENERY: ✿ ✿ ✿ ✿
TRAIL CONDITION: ✿ ✿ ✿
CHILDREN: ✿ ✿ ✿
DIFFICULTY: ✿ ✿
SOLITUDE: ✿ ✿ ✿
DISTANCE: *4.8 miles round-trip*
HIKING TIME: *3:15 round-trip*
OUTSTANDING FEATURES: *views, streamside relaxing spot*

THIS LOOP DIPS OFF THE EASTERN SIDE of Hogback Mountain into the upper Piney River valley. You will enjoy far-reaching views on the Appalachian Trail (AT), then follow a moderate grade into the Piney River on the relatively new Sugarloaf Trail. A grassy flat beside the Piney River makes for a great resting spot. Head back to the high country, grabbing a few more views from Hogback Mountain before completing the loop.

🐾 From the parking area just south of Hogback Overlook, pick up the AT as it crosses over to the eastern side of Skyline Drive. Head northbound through fern-floored woods, shortly climbing to a rocky knob with uptilted rock. Note the rock combination just to the right of the trail that resembles a chair. Many a hiker has had their picture taken in that throne. At 0.2 miles, a side trail leads left to a rock outcrop framed in mountain ash trees. The western vistas are extensive. Descend among rocky woods to reach the Sugarloaf Trail at 0.3 miles. Here, turn right onto a single-track path lined with mountain laurel beneath scattered oaks. Briefly run parallel to Skyline Drive, joining an old wagon road.

The Sugarloaf Trail curves back to the right, descending to cross two rocky streamlets, feeder branches of the Piney River, before reaching a trail junction at mile 1.7. Turn right onto the Pole Bridge Link Trail. The land is level in these parts—for mountain land. It was once cultivated, despite the rocks you see. Pass through a changing forest, where many of the hemlocks here are dead or dying, victim of the woolly adelgid. Reach another trail junction at 2.1 miles and turn right onto the Piney Branch Trail. Step over rocky branches before reaching the upper Piney River in 0.1 mile. Large boulders and rocks line the watercourse. Cross the river to a grassy flat flanked by a large boulder. This locale makes a nice respite.

SUGARLOAF LOOP

Tuscarora Overall Run Trl.

Hogback Overlook

Hogback Mtn.

Little Devils Stairs Overlook

Sugarloaf Trl.

Keyser Run Fire Rd.

Rattlesnake Point Overlook

Piney River

Fourway

Little Devils Stairs Trl.

Piney River Ranger Station

Piney Branch Trl.

cabin

Pole Bridge Link Trl.

Piney Ridge Trl.

Piney River

Piney River Trl.

Keyser Run Fire Rd.

N

0   2000
Feet

ELEVATION PROFILE

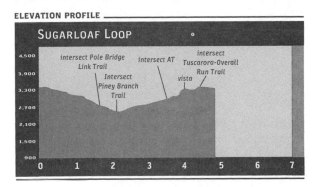

SUGARLOAF LOOP

intersect Pole Bridge Link Trail

intersect AT

intersect Tuscarora-Overall Run Trail

Intersect Piney Branch Trail

vista

4,500
3,900
3,300
2,700
2,100
1,500
900

0   1   2   3   4   5   6   7

Leave this low point of the loop and start climbing toward the crest of the Blue Ridge on a gentle grade. Big rocks line the trailbed. At mile 3.2, pass through an open area with a tremendous rock face up the hill to your right. In September, bears converge here and eat cherries from the cherry trees that grow here. You will see much purple, seed-laden bear scat along the path. Curve uphill away from the roadbed to cross a second roadbed near a national park survey marker. The AT is just uphill, at mile 3.5. Turn right onto the AT, making northbound tracks through open woodland where large widespread oaks grow over grass. Undulate over a rocky hill to reach Skyline Drive at mile 3.8. Rattlesnake Point Overlook is just uproad. Keep northbound, crossing Skyline Drive, and ascend the south side of

Hogback Mountain. A side trail at mile 4 leads left to an outcrop with views of Massanutten Mountain and range upon range of Shenandoah's mountains to the south. Dip into a pretty, grassy gap, then resume climbing to reach the Tuscarora-Overall Run Trail at mile 4.4. Keep forward on the AT drifting into the parking area at mile 4.8, completing your loop.

Directions: From Thornton Gap entrance station, take Skyline Drive north for 10.4 miles to the parking area just before Hogback Mountain Overlook. It will be on your left at milepost 21.1. The loop hike starts on the eastern side of Skyline Drive where the AT crosses Skyline Drive.

Little Devils Stairs Loop

SCENERY: ✪ ✪ ✪ ✪ ✪
DIFFICULTY: ✪ ✪ ✪ ✪
TRAIL CONDITION: ✪ ✪
SOLITUDE: ✪ ✪
CHILDREN: ✪
DISTANCE: *5.8 miles round-trip*
HIKING TIME: *3:45 round-trip*
OUTSTANDING FEATURES: *incredible rugged gorge, big trees, pioneer cemetery*

THIS PHYSICALLY CHALLENGING BUT VISUALLY *rewarding hike gives you something for every step you take. You will undertake the challenging part (heading up Little Devils Stairs Canyon) at the beginning when you are fresh. The water, the rocks, the trees—there is beauty everywhere you look in this canyon. Once you are out of the canyon, cruise down the mountains on the Keyser Run Fire Road, passing the Bolen Cemetery along the way.*

🚶🚶 Leave the Little Devils Stairs parking area on the Little Devils Stairs Trail and immediately cross two small streams. Enter a field and notice the piles of rock. At 0.2 miles Keyser Run comes into view. Turn left and begin to trace the creek up the canyon. At this point the grade is gentle, but the footing is rocky.

At 0.6 miles the trail actually drops to cross a normally dry streambed. You'll soon rock hop Keyser Run on the first of many crossings, all of which should be easy at normal water levels. The canyon becomes narrow and the forest becomes lush. Walk over, around, and among large boulders that litter the canyon floor. Beside you, the stream seeks its way down the gorge as fast as gravity allows.

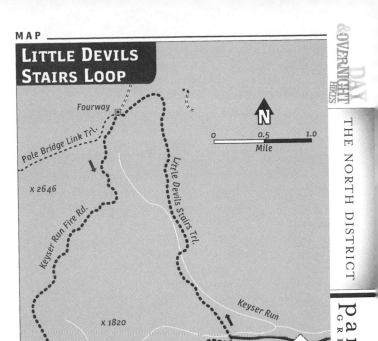

LITTLE DEVILS STAIRS LOOP

Fourway

Pole Bridge Link Trl.

x 2646

Keyser Run Fire Rd.

Little Devils Stairs Trl.

Keyser Run

x 1820

614

Bolen Cemetery

Keyser Run Fire Rd.

N

0   0.5   1.0
Mile

ELEVATION PROFILE

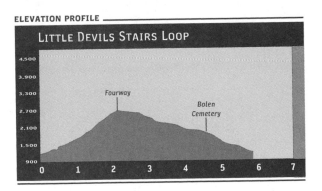

LITTLE DEVILS STAIRS LOOP

Fourway

Bolen Cemetery

Trail and creek merge many times as the sheer walls of the canyon rise straight up around you. Impressive red maple, yellow birch, and tulip trees grow on the rocky soil where they can gain purchase. The trail is very steep here and sometimes hard to follow. Watch for the blue blazes and keep going up. At mile 1.8 make your last crossing of Keyser Run to the left side of the gorge. Soon, the trail switchbacks to the left at a point where you can see the creek spilling over rock in a 15-foot cascade.

Gently climb a series of switchbacks and level off, coming to the Keyser Run Fire Road at mile 2.2. This trail junction is known as Fourway. Turn left on the Keyser Run Fire Road and begin an easy descent after your climb out of the rigorous canyon. Enjoy the forest around you.

At mile 2.6, come to a cleared area beneath a large oak and make a short, steep descent. The trail undulates downward, leveling in an area of white pine at mile 3.7.

Arrive at the Bolen Cemetery at mile 4.6. The well-tended cemetery is lined with red maples and surrounded by a rock wall. The graves range from carved marble to simple field stones. Just beyond is the Hull School Trail. Stay left on the fire road and descend beneath more white pines before coming to a gravel road at mile 5.6. Keep left, walk 0.2 miles farther, and complete your loop at mile 5.8.

Directions: From Thornton Gap, take US 211 east for 7 miles to Sperryville. Continue on US 211 for 2.5 miles past Sperryville to VA 622. Turn left on VA 622 and follow it for 2.1 miles to VA 614. Turn left on VA 614, following it for 3.1 miles as it turns to gravel and ends at the Little Devils Stairs parking area. The Little Devils Stairs Trail leaves the right-hand side of the parking area.

Knob Mountain/
Jeremys Run Loop

SCENERY: ✪ ✪ ✪ ✪ ✪
DIFFICULTY: ✪ ✪ ✪ ✪
TRAIL CONDITION: ✪ ✪ ✪
SOLITUDE: ✪ ✪ ✪
CHILDREN: ✪
DISTANCE: *12.1 miles round-trip*
HIKING TIME: *8:00 round-trip*
OUTSTANDING FEATURES: *good views, intimate stream valley, quality trout fishing*

THIS IS A LONG, YET REWARDING, LOOP. *Leave the Appalachian Trail (AT) and traverse the ridgeline of Knob Mountain, enjoying views on the way to Jeremys Run. Make your way up the valley of Jeremys Run, crossing the stream more than a dozen times. Watch for brook trout as you pass the many deep pools*

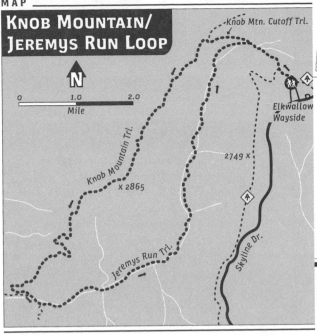

KNOB MOUNTAIN/ JEREMYS RUN LOOP

0   1.0   2.0
Mile

Knob Mtn. Cutoff Trl.

Elkwallow Wayside

2749 x

x 2865

Knob Mountain Trl.

Jeremys Run Trl.

Skyline Dr.

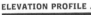

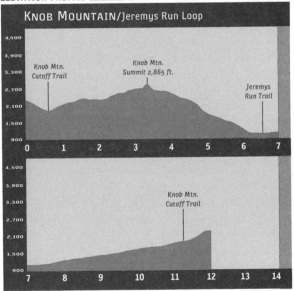

in Jeremys Run. Leave the valley and return to the high country. Don't expect to have company on Knob Mountain, though you may see a few people along Jeremys Run.

🚶 Start your loop on the spur trail that goes from the low end of the Elkwallow Picnic Area to intersect the AT in 50 yards. Veer left onto the AT and head downhill through a forest carpeted with grass in the summer. Pass a marked spring on your left and come to Jeremys Run Trail at 0.2 miles.

Continue forward on Jeremys Run Trail. Switchback downward to parallel Jeremys Run before meeting Knob Mountain Cutoff Trail at 0.7 miles, crossing an intermittent stream on the way. Turn right on Knob Mountain Cutoff Trail and immediately cross Jeremys Run. Get water here, because there is none for miles along Knob Mountain.

After crossing Jeremys Run, the trail switchbacks to the left and begins heading west toward Knob Mountain. The trail, which is on a steep grade that makes use of a few old roads, levels off and reaches Knob Mountain Trail at mile 1.2. Turn left on Knob Mountain Trail, following a former fire road. Here, the trail undulates over small prominences and outcrops and then dips into gaps, climbing ever so slightly toward the Knob Mountain summit. Views of the Shenandoah Valley are to your right.

There is no tree canopy over much of the trail. The forest is recovering from gypsy-moth damage and will grow thicker in the future. By mile 3 the ridge becomes wide and level. This is grouse country; don't be surprised if a brown fowl flutters away from your feet. Just before reaching the summit, the former fire road ends at a concrete post. Continue forward on a footpath, making an abrupt ascent to the summit (2,865 feet) at mile 3.4.

The trail drops sharply from the summit. Look through the trees for Massanutten Mountain and the town of Luray as you work your way toward Jeremys Run. The path makes repeated switchbacks on the ridge. At mile 4.6 the trail crosses a gap and traces the left side of the ridge. Jeremys Run lies below and Neighbor Mountain is across the valley. More switchbacks with great views of the Shenandoah Valley lead through an area of pine trees. Pass a spring on your right at mile 5.9.

Soon the intonations of Jeremys Run can be heard. At mile 6.7, cross the creek at the head of a large pool and turn left onto Jeremys Run Trail. Just ahead is the Neighbor Mountain Trail junction where you'll find some good rocks for taking a break.

Start up Jeremys Run Trail on a mild grade, passing a small cascade on your right at mile 7.3.

Stone walls line the path. White pines now grow on former fields, while sycamores shade the stream where brook trout gather in deep pools.

When rock bluffs crowd the stream, the trail crosses to the other side toward flatter terrain. This pattern of crowding and crossing continues up the valley. In times of high water these fords will become dangerous, but most of the time you can make it dry-shod.

At mile 10.4 the trail appears to end on a mud bluff overlooking the creek. Here the trail has been washed out from a flood. Continue carefully along the bluff and pick up the trail in 40 feet. More crossings bring you to the head of the valley and the junction with Knob Mountain Cutoff Trail at mile 11.4.

Bear right and retrace your steps up Jeremys Run Trail for 0.5 miles, coming once again to the AT. Go straight, head up the AT for 0.2 mile, and veer right onto the spur trail to the Elkwallow Picnic Area, completing your loop at mile 12.1.

> **Directions: From Thornton Gap, take Skyline Drive north for 7.4 miles to Elkwallow Wayside at milepost 24.1. Drive to the low end of the picnic area and park. The spur trail to the AT leaves here.**

Broad Hollow/*Pine Hill Gap Loop*

SCENERY: ☆ ☆ ☆
TRAIL CONDITION: ☆ ☆
CHILDREN: ☆ ☆
DIFFICULTY: ☆ ☆ ☆
SOLITUDE: ☆ ☆ ☆ ☆
DISTANCE: *5.8 miles round-trip*
HIKING TIME: *4:15 round-trip*
OUTSTANDING FEATURES: *Homesites, wooden cabin, views*

THIS IS A CHALLENGING LOOP STARTING *at a lesser-used trailhead. The two primary trails used, Broad Hollow Trail and Pine Hill Gap Trail, are both steep. The area between the two paths, on the flank of Hazel Mountain, is mostly level. The fires of the year 2000 left their mark in this slice of "Hazel River Country," which was heavily settled. As you ascend Broad Hollow, you wonder how someone desired to farm such hilly terrain.*

🚶 Start your loop hike by looking for the park boundary signs and the blue-blazed trail leading beside a residence. Pick up the Broad Hollow Trail,

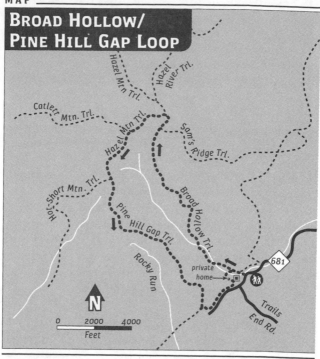

BROAD HOLLOW/ PINE HILL GAP LOOP

Hazel Mtn. Trl.

Hazel River Trl.

Catlett Mtn. Trl.

Hazel Mtn. Trl.

Sam's Ridge Trl.

Hot-Short Mtn. Trl.

Pine Hill Gap Trl.

Broad Hollow Trl.

Rocky Run

private home →

681

Trails End Rd.

N

0   2000   4000
Feet

ELEVATION PROFILE

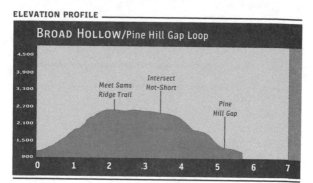

BROAD HOLLOW/Pine Hill Gap Loop

Meet Sams Ridge Trail

Intersect Hot-Short

Pine Hill Gap

passing a concrete trail post just beyond the rock hop over the stream forming Broad Hollow. Keep the farmstead to your left as you head upstream in woods recovering from fire.

Leave the farmstead behind and again rock hop the stream of Broad Hollow at 0.3 miles. Broad Hollow is anything but broad at this point. Look around and you will see piled rocks, evidence of previous tilling. It has been said that Appalachian farmers plowed slopes so steep they could "hoe corn on their knees." Rock fences run through the hollow on the far side of the branch. Moisture loving trees occupy the valley nowadays, such as tulip trees, sweet birch, sugar maple, and even a few yellow birches, which like cool, damp places.

Cross back over the stream at 0.5 miles. Typical of Shenandoah's streams, this watercourse can range from a trickle to a torrent, depending on rainfall and the time of year. When the water is up, cascades will abound; when the water is low, you will barely get your feet wet. The stream can generally be rock hopped in all but the strongest of flows.

The trail steepens, passing more rock walls and the rock foundations of a cabin downhill to your left. The woods are more open here. Look for scattered large trees. At mile 1.1, pass directly by a rocked-in spring on your right. Ahead, just uphill, is an old wooden cabin. Notice the wood shingles on the outside of the roofless structure. The trail leaves the hollow for open mountainside. Brush is growing thick among the scattered trees. Top out among mountain laurel and hemlock skeletons before mildly dipping to reach the Sams Ridge Trail at mile 2.2. Turn left here and run through level land, in conjunction with the Sams Ridge Trail, to make a second junction at mile 2.4.

Turn left on the yellow-blazed Hazel Mountain Trail. The walking remains easy on the wide path and meets the Catlett Mountain Trail at mile 2.9. Stay left, still on the Hazel Mountain Trail. Many white pines thrive here. At mile 3.4, the Hot-Short Mountain Trail leaves right. Stay forward, now on the infrequently trod Pine Hill Gap Trail. Dip over to the right-hand side of the ridge and begin an extended descent, passing an abandoned trail, still marked by a concrete trail post at mile 3.7. The abandoned trail leads to Hot Mountain.

Views open to the right, a by-product of previous fires, but they will close as the forest recovers. The trailbed becomes rocky and begins to drop steeply. Be glad you are going downhill. Pass a rock wall in Pine Hill Gap at mile 5.2. Skirt the park boundary, splitting left at mile 5.4. Descend an eroded old road lined with rock walls, emerging onto the gated portion of VA 681. Keep forward on the road, passing Trails End Road and the bus turnaround parking area to complete your loop at mile 5.7.

Directions: From Thornton Gap on Skyline Drive, head east on US 211 for 7 miles to US 522 south, Sperryville Pike. Follow US 522 south for 0.7 miles to VA 231. Turn right on

VA 231 and follow it for 3.3 miles to VA 681, Rolling Road, just before VA 231 crosses the Hazel River. Turn right onto VA 681 and follow it for 2.5 miles to the Broad Hollow Trail on your right, beside a home on a left curve. Parking is limited here to the two spaces located on the curve. Do not block the private driveway. On weekends, however, you can park at a school-bus turnaround about 100 yards up the road, on the left. Do not park at the turnaround on school days.

Buck Ridge/*Buck Hollow Loop*

SCENERY: ✿ ✿ ✿ ✿
DIFFICULTY: ✿ ✿ ✿
TRAIL CONDITION: ✿ ✿ ✿
SOLITUDE: ✿ ✿ ✿ ✿ ✿
CHILDREN: ✿
DISTANCE: *5.8 miles round-trip*
HIKING TIME: *3:45 round-trip*
OUTSTANDING FEATURES: *big trees, some views, isolation*

ENJOY BOTH RIDGETOP AND RIVERINE *environments on this loop. Start down Hazel Mountain and then traverse the narrow Buck Ridge Trail. Some views open up before the path dives steeply from the side of the ridge down to Buck Hollow. Look for signs of human habitation as you encounter a series of old roads in the valley. Except during June, July, and October weekends, you should have this little-used gem to yourself.*

🚶🚶 Begin the hike by descending the Hazel Mountain Trail. The gated fire road drops to a small clearing at 0.3 miles before coming to the junction with Buck Ridge Trail at 0.5 miles. Turn left on the hemlock-lined Buck Ridge Trail as it hugs the right side of Buck Ridge.

As the trail turns southward, the forest changes character; lichen-covered chestnut oaks tower over mountain laurel. Notice the preponderance of sassafras, a small understory tree with mitten-shaped leaves. Scratch a twig and smell the sweet aroma. Sassafras roots, used to flavor root beer, were one of Colonial America's first exports.

At mile 1.4, the trail drops steeply among ridgetop boulders. Intermittent views of Pass Mountain open up on the left. At mile 1.7 a spur trail to the right leads to views of the Hazel River area. Here, the trail's grade moderates as it takes a northward tack and then swings below an outcrop with more views to the left.

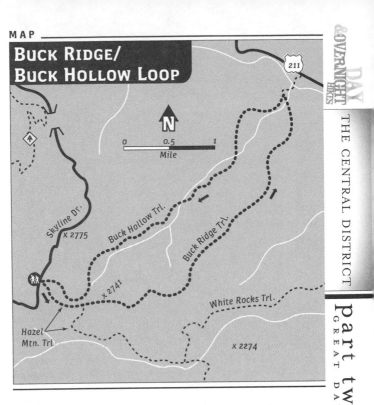

ELEVATION PROFILE

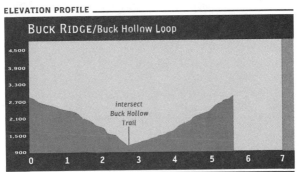

At mile 2.3 Buck Ridge Trail takes a nosedive toward Buck Hollow. In some places the trail is so steep that log steps have been installed to provide better footing, though the descent can be hard on the knees. At mile 2.7 this leg-jarring descent ends, and the trail follows an old road to cross the watercourse forming Buck Hollow. Just beyond the rock hop across the water is the Buck Hollow Trail at mile 2.8.

Turn left and walk up the rocky, wooded road that is Buck Hollow Trail. Cross the creek once again at mile 3 and continue up the moist valley. The dense forest consists of beech, birch, maple, and assorted oaks. The stream can always be heard, if not seen, along this stretch of trail.

Rock hop the stream, again, at mile 3.6 onto a trail that is now a narrow footpath. Buck Hollow has narrowed, too. At mile 3.9 the trail turns away from the stream and climbs among sizeable red oak, hickory, and tulip trees. Unfortunately, there are large skeletons of hemlocks that fell prey to the woolly adelgid. Again the trail nears the stream, passing three small but attractive cascades.

Cross the stream for the last time and continue climbing. The upper end of the hollow flattens out. On the final push, Buck Hollow Trail passes through a grassy area, completing the loop at mile 5.6.

Directions: From Thornton Gap, take Skyline Drive south for 2 miles to the Meadow Spring parking area at milepost 33.5. The parking area is on the left side of Skyline Drive.

Hazeltop/*Rapidan Camp Loop*

SCENERY: ✿ ✿ ✿ ✿
DIFFICULTY: ✿ ✿
TRAIL CONDITION: ✿ ✿ ✿ ✿
SOLITUDE: ✿ ✿
CHILDREN: ✿ ✿ ✿
DISTANCE: *7.2 miles round-trip*
HIKING TIME: *6:00 round-trip (includes 1 hour at Rapidan Camp)*
OUTSTANDING FEATURES: *Rapidan Camp, Big Rock Falls*

THIS LOOP TAKES YOU OVER HAZELTOP, *the third highest peak in the park, and then traces the attractive Laurel Prong Trail down to Rapidan Camp, once known as Camp Hoover, the woodland getaway for President Herbert Hoover (1929–33). Rapidan Camp has much to see; you can even embark on a self-guided interpretive tour. Return to Milam Gap via Mill Prong Trail and view Big Rock Falls along the way.*

🚶 Head southbound on the Appalachian Trail (AT) from the Milam Gap parking area. Cross Skyline Drive and come to a trail junction. To your left is Mill Prong Trail (your return route). Continue southbound on the AT through a forest, shading fields of ferns, and reach a sharp right turn at mile 0.4. Now you are really going south as the AT heads toward Hazeltop.

HAZELTOP/RAPIDAN CAMP LOOP

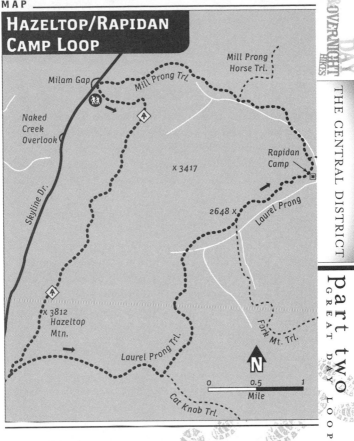

ELEVATION PROFILE

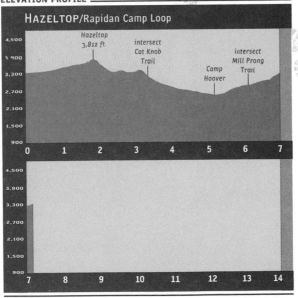

The trail grade is nearly level, but it rises slightly on a slowly narrowing ridge to achieve the summit of Hazeltop (3,812 feet) at mile 1.9. To your right is a gnarled oak next to a large embedded rock (the top of the summit). To the left of the trail is a small balsam fir, a survivor of the forests that now thrive much farther north in New England and Canada. Its needles are flat, fragrant, and friendly (not sharp). Leave the summit and come to a left turn. To your right are two red spruce trees, another member of the Canadian forest. Its needles are a darker green, rounded, and sharp. These trees grow only in a few locations in the park.

The AT drops moderately and approaches the scenic Laurel Prong Trail at mile 2.4. Turn left on Laurel Prong Trail and pass several springs on a boulder-laden slope. The trail descends sharply just before arriving at Laurel Gap and another trail junction at mile 3.4. Turn left, staying on the Laurel Prong Trail, which continues to drop sharply until it comes to a dark hemlock thicket at mile 3.9. The trail levels off here.

Amid many downed trees, the path crosses several rills flowing off Hazeltop. At mile 4.7, Fork Mountain Trail appears to your right. Continue forward on the Laurel Prong Trail, nearing a road junction. Veer right and arrive at Rapidan Camp at mile 5.2. At the confluence of Laurel Prong and Mill Creek, Rapidan Camp lies in a lovely wooded setting. Walk around, check out the buildings and interpretive signs. There are short nature trails here, too. This place is engaging, so give it at least an hour.

Continue your loop hike on the Mill Prong Trail, which starts near The Creel Cabin. Climb along the steep Mill Prong Trail. Look for an old building along the creek at mile 5.4. The trail now drops to Mill Prong, crossing it below Big Rock Falls at mile 5.6. Big Rock Falls is wide, spilling 15 or 20 feet into a large pool that Herbert Hoover surely fished.

The trail switchbacks, levels off, and intersects the Mill Prong Horse Trail at mile 6.2. Bear left on the Mill Prong Trail, crossing a side branch, and then rock hop Mill Prong once more at mile 6.6. The trail leads back into an open, fern forest and enters a grassy glade before intersecting the AT at mile 7.2. Turn right on the AT, cross Skyline Drive, and return to Milam Gap.

Directions: From Swift Run Gap, drive north on Skyline Drive for 12.7 miles to Milam Gap (mile 53). The AT is accessible right behind the parking area. Start your hike here.

Rocky Mount Loop

SCENERY: ✿ ✿ ✿ ✿
DIFFICULTY: ✿ ✿ ✿ ✿
TRAIL CONDITION: ✿ ✿ ✿
SOLITUDE: ✿ ✿ ✿ ✿ ✿
CHILDREN: ✿
DISTANCE: *9.8 miles round-trip*
HIKING TIME: *6:00 round-trip*
OUTSTANDING FEATURES: *Solitude, views from Rocky Mount*

IF YOU LIKE WILDERNESS HIKING IN SOLITUDE, *take this ambitious loop. Leave the main crest of the Blue Ridge to access the summit of Rocky Mount for far-reaching views. Descend sharply to Gap Run and return up the watershed to the Rocky Mount Trail. You'll have this untamed slice of Shenandoah to yourself.*

🐾 Head north from Skyline Drive on Rocky Mount Trail and briefly climb a knoll before heading northeast on a narrow ridge. The trail alternately dips and levels off before coming to a saddle at 0.7 miles. Veer to the left side of the ridge among pine woods. To your left are intermittent views of Rocky Mountain (not to be confused with Rocky Mount).

At 1.1 mile come to a gap and swing around the north end of an unnamed knob. The forest changes to birch trees with a high canopy. Descend to another gap and a trail junction at mile 2.2. To your right is Gap Run Trail, your return route. Continue on Rocky Mount Trail, climbing the south face of Rocky Mount.

Cross a talus slope at mile 2.6 and then switchback. Twice you'll think you're nearing the summit, but the trail keeps rising. Come to a side trail on your left just before reaching the true summit of Rocky Mount (2,741 feet) at mile 3.3. This leads to an outcrop with stunning views. Look over Two Mile Run. At the head of the run is the Two Mile Run Overlook, where you started, and the crest of the Blue Ridge. To your right is the Shenandoah Valley.

Beyond the wooded summit, the trail drops along the base of a huge granite slope. Continue descending through a heavily canopied forest before coming to a pine stand with views into Gap Run. On

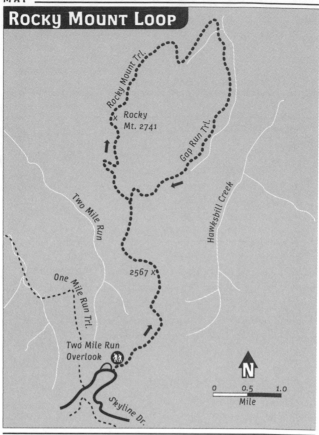

ROCKY MOUNT LOOP

Rocky Mount Trl.

Rocky Mt. 2741

Gap Run Trl.

Two Mile Run

Hawksbill Creek

One Mile Run Trl.

2567 X

Two Mile Run Overlook

Skyline Dr.

N

0   0.5   1.0
Mile

a switchback the rocky slope of Beldor Ridge is visible directly ahead. Traverse a rock field at mile 4.6 and follow a tributary of Gap Run, crossing it twice in succession. Make a sharp right turn into a clearing before rock hopping Gap Run and come to a trail junction at mile 5.3.

Turn right on Gap Run Trail, gently ascending on an old road that has been washed out in places. Pass through a clearing and come to a second trail marker at mile 5.5. There is a real aura of isolation here, even though this valley was once peopled.

Stay on the roadbed and enter the rock-strewn flood plain of Gap Run. Look for a cairn marking the path and pick up the roadbed again, coming to another trail marker at mile 6.1. Turn right and travel along Gap Run, crossing the creek easily three times and leaving the roadbed behind.

After the last ford, the trail grade sharpens and Gap Run follows a dry wash toward a low spot on

ELEVATION PROFILE

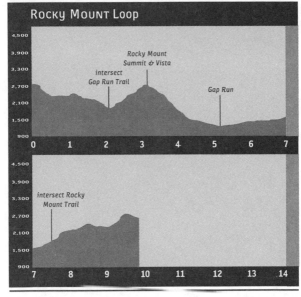

Rocky Mount Loop

Rocky Mount Summit & Vista

intersect Gap Run Trail

Gap Run

intersect Rocky Mount Trail

Rocky Mount Trail. Leave the dry wash at a switch-back and surge upward on the trail a short distance, reaching the gap at mile 7.6. Turn left on Rocky Mount Trail and retrace your steps 2.2 miles back to Skyline Drive and the Blue Ridge.

Directions: From Swift Run Gap drive south on Skyline Drive for 10.7 miles to Two Mile Run Overlook (mile 76.2), which will be on your right. Hike back north 0.1 mile on Skyline Drive to Rocky Mount Trail.

Loft Mountain Loop

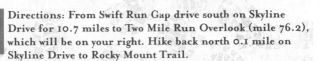

SCENERY: ✿ ✿ ✿ ✿
TRAIL CONDITION: ✿ ✿ ✿ ✿
CHILDREN: ✿ ✿ ✿ ✿
DIFFICULTY: ✿ ✿
SOLITUDE: ✿
DISTANCE: *3 miles round-trip*
HIKING TIME: *1:45 round-trip*
OUTSTANDING FEATURES: *views from big rock outcrop, camp store*

THIS LOOP IS IDEAL FOR A FAMILY HIKE *or just an afternoon stroll. Start at the Loft Mountain Wayside and take the Frazier Discovery Trail to a massive rock outcrop with an extensive view. Beyond the vista, pick up the world's most famous footpath, the Appalachian Trail (AT), southward through a transitional forest to*

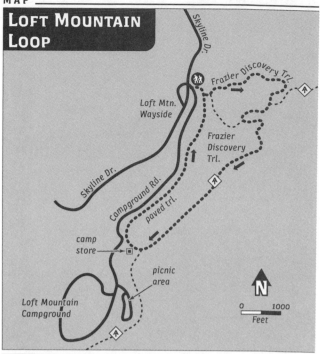

LOFT MOUNTAIN LOOP

Skyline Dr.

Frazier Discovery Trl.

Loft Mtn. Wayside

Frazier Discovery Trl.

Skyline Dr.

Campground Rd.

paved trl.

camp store

picnic area

Loft Mountain Campground

N

0   1000
Feet

ELEVATION PROFILE

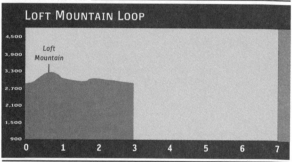

LOFT MOUNTAIN LOOP

4,500

Loft
Mountain

3,900

3,300

2,700

2,100

1,500

900

0   1   2   3   4   5   6   7

meet a paved path near the Loft Mountain Campground camp store. Gently descend back to Loft Mountain Wayside. The hike is easy, though the first part does climb to the rock outcrop.

🚶 Leave the Loft Mountain Wayside and cross Skyline Drive. Begin climbing up a paved path that is now as much gravel and moss as pavement. Shortly intersect the Frazier Discovery Trail, turning left. Where the dirt path splits; stay left again, and head uphill on a rocky slope. Before 1999, this trail was known as the "Deadening Trail," named after the settler practice of girding trees. This practice killed the trees but left them standing, preventing the leaves from blocking crucial sunlight for crops. All evidence of tree deadening has disintegrated with time, and the trail name was changed. Curve beneath a big rock overhang and keep climbing to a rock outcrop jutting into the sky at 0.6 miles. Enjoy the panoramic view from 3,300 feet atop Loft Mountain. To your west are many peaks of Shenandoah National Park, the Shenandoah Valley and the Alleghenies of West Virginia in the hazy distance. Floyd Frazier called this outcrop "Raven Rocks." He and his family lived below the outcrop in pre-park days. The Frazier clan tended cattle for the owners of the land in exchange for squatter's rights. Loft Mountain was previously known as Frazier Mountain and Lost Mountain.

Leave the rocky vista and join the AT, heading southbound along the Frazier Discovery Trail. Soon, a side trail leading right opens to a second vista. Ahead, stay on the AT as the Frazier Discovery Trail leaves right. Many spindly, narrow-trunked trees crowd the AT through here. Locust and cherry trees indicate recent reforestation. This was likely once pastureland where Frazier tended cattle. Look for larger oak trees with widespread limbs amid the younger trees. The limbs on these older trees, that once enjoyed sunlight, are now denied light as a result of reforestation, and some limbs are dying and breaking off. Parts of the trail pass through low brushy areas open to the sky.

Keep forward, again on the AT, and pass a rough road leading 0.5 miles to the camp store. The trailbed becomes grassy and at 1.8 miles, turn right on a narrow trail leading 75 yards to the Loft Mountain camp store—a rarity so close to the trail. This turn is marked with a concrete post. Pass behind the camp store and take advantage of its offerings if you are hungry or thirsty. Just past the store, turn right onto an unnamed paved trail. Gently descend on the crumbly path beneath hawthorn and locust trees, trees that typically reclaim old fields. Look on trail left for a water fountain made to appear as if the spigot is coming directly from the rock. Trailside fountains are about as rare as trailside camp stores. Shortly pass the Frazier Discovery Trail a final time before reaching Loft Mountain Wayside at 3 miles, ending your loop.

Directions: From Rockfish Gap entrance station, take Skyline Drive 26.1 miles north to Loft Mountain Wayside, mile 79.5, on the left. The Frazier Discovery Trail leaves from the wayside near the entrance to Loft Mountain Campground.

Falls Loop *from Browns Gap*

> SCENERY: ✩ ✩ ✩ ✩ ✩
>
> DIFFICULTY: ✩ ✩
>
> TRAIL CONDITION: ✩ ✩ ✩ ✩
>
> SOLITUDE: ✩ ✩
>
> CHILDREN: ✩ ✩ ✩
>
> DISTANCE: *6.6 miles round-trip*
>
> HIKING TIME: *4:15 round-trip*
>
> OUTSTANDING FEATURES: *waterfalls, cascades, large trees*

WATER LOVERS WILL FALL FOR THIS LOOP. *The trail passes three major falls and numerous other cascades as it explores two boulder-strewn canyons and incorporates one section of the Appalachian Trail (AT). The hike up Jones Run passes some old-growth tulip trees with impressive girths, and the trail grades are generally moderate. Add a little human history, and you have a great loop hike.*

The hike starts at Browns Gap, a location of historical significance. Stonewall Jackson passed through here in early 1862 while outwitting Union forces in the Shenandoah Mountains. The Union later defended the gap because of the strategic turnpike, which was built in 1805, connecting Richmond with the Shenandoah Valley.

Cross Skyline Drive and immediately begin descending on the Browns Gap Fire Road, the same road of yore. Look for a small path leaving the road to your left at mile 0.4. Scramble a few feet up this path to the grave of William H. Howard, Confederate States of America soldier. Return to the fire road and continue down the trail on a gentle grade, passing through a stand of pines.

On your left at 0.9 miles, a cleared area containing relics indicates former human habitation. As the trail swings to the left, the canopy of tulip trees and oaks thickens. Cross an iron bridge spanning normally short and shallow Doyles River and reach a trail junction at mile 1.8.

Turn right onto Doyles River Trail. The footpath descends and crosses Doyles River on an easy rock hop at mile 1.9. Notice all the dead hemlocks here. They are under attack by an invasive insect known as the woolly adelgid, which kills these trees by sucking the sap out of them. The wooly adelgid is thought to have been introduced to the U.S. from Asia in 1924. It is feared that most hemlocks in the park will succumb to this deadly pest.

THE SOUTH DISTRICT

part two
GREAT DAY LOOPS

DAY
&OVERNIGHT
HIKES

MAP

FALLS LOOP

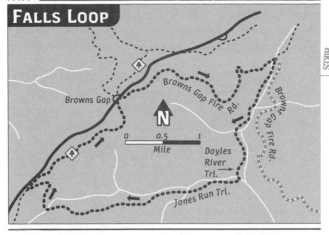

Browns Gap

Browns Gap Fire Rd.

Browns Gap Fire Rd.

N

0   0.5   1
Mile

Doyles River Trl.

Jones Run Trl.

ELEVATION PROFILE

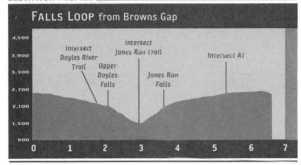

FALLS LOOP from Browns Gap

intersect Doyles River Trail

intersect Jones Run Trail

Upper Doyles Falls

Jones Run Falls

intersect AT

Doyles River Trail continues along the watercourse but swings away as it approaches Upper Doyles Falls. At mile 2.1 a side trail leads to the dark pool at the base of the three-tiered falls. Many unnamed cascades accompany you downstream until a sharp switchback leads you to the base of Lower Doyles Falls at mile 2.4. Lower Doyles Falls is the steeper of the two.

The trail squeezes down the narrow gorge, using a wooden bridge to span a cascading branch that spills into Doyles River at mile 2.6. In a small flat that would make a good lunch spot, find a trail junction and the end of Doyles River Trail at mile 3.

Veer right on Jones Run Trail and begin to climb, rock hopping Jones Run at mile 3.1. Here is where you will begin to see some impressive tulip trees. Look up the slope. The Jones Run gorge is littered with huge boulders. Keep an eye on the creek, too, as many scenic cascades tumble down the rocky watercourse. At mile 3.7, you'll arrive at Jones Run Falls, where water spills 50 feet over a solid rock wall.

The trail turns sharply left, and then right, to achieve the top of the falls. It traces Jones Run for a short distance before veering away from the creek. Gently ascend through a cove-hardwood forest with an open understory of grass and ferns.

At mile 4.8, cross Jones Run, which is minute at this point. The trail begins to ascend more steeply and arrives at the AT at mile 5.4. Turn right on the AT and head north. The grade back to Browns Gap is very gentle, with intermittent mountain views opening up to your right. The AT descends before arriving at Browns Gap and completing your loop at mile 6.6.

Directions: From the Rockfish Gap entrance station take Skyline Drive north for 21.6 miles to Browns Gap parking area (milepost 83), which will be on your left.

Turk Branch Loop

SCENERY: ☆ ☆ ☆ ☆
TRAIL CONDITION: ☆ ☆ ☆
CHILDREN: ☆ ☆
DIFFICULTY: ☆ ☆ ☆
SOLITUDE: ☆ ☆ ☆ ☆
DISTANCE: *7.5 miles round-trip*
HIKING TIME: *4:00 round-trip*
OUTSTANDING FEATURES: *old homesites, some views, solitude*

THIS LOOP TRAVERSES THE PARK'S *most southerly and seemingly most forgotten reaches. Leave the crest of the Blue Ridge and drop down along Turk Branch, passing old homesites where Turk Branch meets the South Fork of the Moormans River. Head up the uppermost part of the rocky South Fork valley to meet the Appalachian Trail (AT). Head north on Shenandoah's master path, gaining views amid the pines and oaks before returning to Turk Gap. Though the elevation change is nearly 1,000 feet, the trail grades are never sharp.*

🚶 The hardest part of the loop may be finding its beginning. Don't take the unmarked trail at the east end of the parking lot; instead, look for the concrete post directly beside Skyline Drive just south of the Turk Gap parking area. Head past the post to trace an old roadbed running parallel to Skyline Drive. You'll know you're on the right track when you see yellow blazes leading downhill through an oak-dominated forest. At 0.3 miles, the Turk

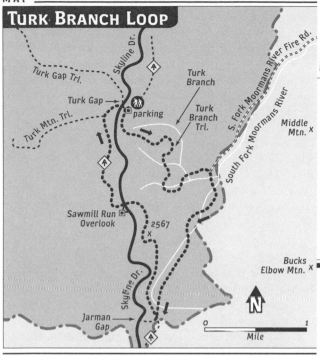

TURK BRANCH LOOP

Turk Gap Trl.

Skyline Dr.

Turk Gap →

parking

Turk Mtn. Trl.

Turk Branch

Turk Branch Trl.

S. Fork Moormans River Fire Rd.

S. Fork Moormans River

South Fork Moormans River

Middle Mtn. x

Sawmill Run Overlook

2567 X

Bucks Elbow Mtn. x

Skyline Dr.

Jarman Gap →

N

0   1
Mile

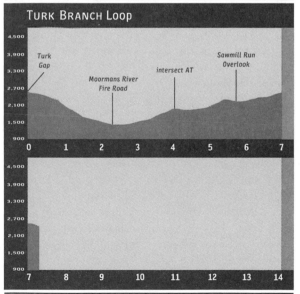

TURK BRANCH LOOP

4,500
3,900
3,300
2,700
2,100
1,500
900

Turk Gap

Moormans River Fire Road

intersect AT

Sawmill Run Overlook

0   1   2   3   4   5   6   7

4,500
3,900
3,300
2,700
2,100
1,500
900

7   8   9   10   11   12   13   14

Branch Trail leads east, away from Skyline Drive.
Descend through a dry ridgeline heavy with mountain laurel and pines. Drop off the ridgeline and
curve down to cross upper Turk Branch at 1.2 miles.

Push over a rib ridge to cross a feeder branch of Turk Branch. Notice the old stonework used to prevent the roadbed from washing away as it crosses the feeder branch at miles 1.7 and 1.9. The trail soon crosses Turk Branch. A small fall cascades above the Turk Branch crossing. Continuing, the Turk Branch valley widens. Piled stones and leveled land indicate a former homesite to the left of the trail. At mile 2.4, approach a survey marker embedded into a boulder marking the junction with the South Fork Moormans River Fire Road. Turn right here, stepping over Turk Branch, and ascend briefly to step over the South Fork of the Moormans River, which is but a small creek at this point. Pass a second homesite to the left of the trail, marked by rock walls, a clearing, a crumbling chimney, and metal relics.

The grade steepens as the hollow pinches in beyond the homesite. At mile 3, again cross the South Fork of the Moormans River. Next, cross a gas line clearing, then what's left of the Moormans River one more time before intersecting the AT at mile 4.1. Turn right here, heading northbound on the AT, dipping along the South Fork of the Moormans River one last time before ascending the east flank of the Blue Ridge, gaining views of Bucks Elbow Mountain across the Moormans River valley. Climb more and cross the gas line clearing again. Views soon open to the south, then west as the AT levels off by mile 5.3. Sawmill Ridge and Turk Mountain can be seen in the distance to the west.

Descend from a high point through brushy woods open overhead to cross Skyline Drive and reach Sawmill Run Overlook at mile 5.7. A picnic table invites hikers to take a break. Begin climbing beyond Skyline Drive and curve past a side trail that leads left through tangled woods to a spring. Level off, then undulate along the path lined with blueberry bushes and mountain laurel. This section of the AT makes for pleasant hiking with no extensive elevation changes through here. Intersect the Turk Mountain Trail at mile 7.1. Keep north on the AT and dip through some pines to emerge at Turk Gap at mile 7.3 and the end of your loop hike.

Directions: From Rockfish Gap entrance station, take Skyline Drive north for 10.5 miles to Turk Gap parking area, milepost 94.3, on your right.

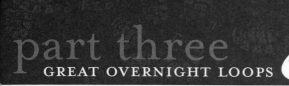

part three
GREAT OVERNIGHT LOOPS

3

The return trip to the AT will get you huffing and puffing, while thinking of all the people that skipped this second view as is evidenced by the much less used trail tread.

Mount Marshall

SCENERY: ✿ ✿ ✿ ✿
TRAIL CONDITION: ✿ ✿
CHILDREN: ✿ ✿
DIFFICULTY: ✿ ✿ ✿
SOLITUDE: ✿ ✿ ✿
DISTANCE: *Day One, 3.6 miles; Day 2, 3.6 miles; Day 3, 6.1 miles*
HIKING TIME: *2:45, 2:30, and 4:00 hours*
OUTSTANDING FEATURES: *Big Devils Stairs, many views, large trees*

THIS OVERNIGHT LOOP CIRCLES *the high country over and around Mount Marshall, staying above 2,000 feet almost its entire length. Start in a gap between North and South Mount Marshall, enjoying some first-rate views on the Appalachian Trail (AT) before dropping off the main crest at Gravel Springs Gap. Here, pass an AT thru-hikers hut before pushing on to the area of the Big Devils Stairs. Your second day is short, as you cruise the east flank of Mount Marshall on a trail that's as level as you can find in this park. Rejoin the AT on your final day and make the pull over North Marshall, where jagged cliffs offer long vistas. The short distances of the first two days allow for side trips, especially along the Big Devils Stairs.*

🚶🚶 DAY 1 Begin your hike by heading south-bound on the AT. The AT immediately crosses Skyline Drive and begins a moderate ascent through brushy hardwoods, anticlimactically topping out on South Mount Marshall at 0.6 miles. Begin descending and look for a side trail leading right to an outcrop over-looking the Shenandoah Valley, Hogback Mountain, Mathews Arm, and Massanutten Mountain. A second view lies a short piece down the AT. Pass a national park service marker at mile 1.3, before reaching Gravel Springs Gap at mile 1.6. Cross Skyline Drive and keep south on the AT, intersecting the Bluff Trail at 1.7 miles. Turn left on the Bluff Trail, switchbacking downhill for 0.3 miles to emerge at Gravel Springs Hut. Gravel Spring is in front of you. This trail shel-ter, maintained by the Potomac Appalachian Trail Club, is for long-distance AT hikers only. Turn left at the concrete trail post and continue along the Bluff Trail. Stay with the Bluff Trail as the Harris Hollow Trail comes in from the right, then leaves left at a sep-arate junction. The Bluff Trail now runs nearly level along the southeast slope of Mount Marshall.

Mount Marshall was named after John Marshall, the longest running chief justice of the United States Supreme Court. Marshall, who served as chief justice

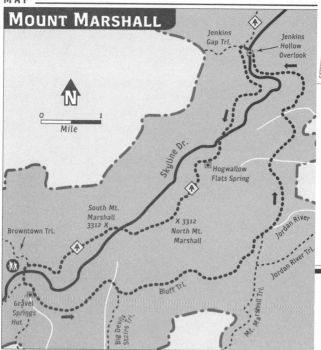

Mount Marshall map — Jenkins Gap Trl., Jenkins Hollow Overlook, Skyline Dr., Hogwallow Flats Spring, South Mt. Marshall 3312 X, X 3312 North Mt. Marshall, Browntown Trl., Bluff Trl., Gravel Springs Hut, Big Devils Stairs Trl., Mt. Marshall Trl., Jordan River, Jordan River Trl. Scale: 0–1 Mile. N.

ELEVATION PROFILE

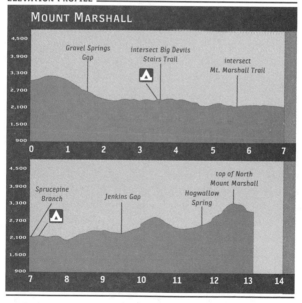

MOUNT MARSHALL

Upper profile (miles 0–7): Gravel Springs Gap; intersect Big Devils Stairs Trail; intersect Mt. Marshall Trail. Elevation axis: 900, 1,500, 2,100, 2,700, 3,300, 3,900, 4,500.

Lower profile (miles 7–14): Sprucepine Branch; Jenkins Gap; Hogwallow Spring; top of North Mount Marshall. Elevation axis: 900, 1,500, 2,100, 2,700, 3,300, 3,900, 4,500.

from 1801 to 1835, owned vast tracts of land in the Blue Ridge.

Continue as large boulders break up the hardwood forest, and many small streamlets cross the trail. Most streams will be dry in late summer and fall.

Make the upper reaches of the Big Devils Stairs gorge at mile 3.6. Rock hop the gorge stream, which is usually flowing, then shortly reach the Big Devils Stairs Trail. Begin looking for a campsite in the next mile or so, on either the Bluff Trail or off the Big Devils Stairs Trail. Good views await 0.7 miles down Big Devils Stairs Trail. A hike down the Big Devils Stairs Trail, then a rock scramble directly up the gorge, is a very worthwhile side trip. The Big Devils Stairs Trail once ran directly up the gorge, but repeated washout necessitated a reroute. The trail now runs along the edge of the gorge.

🏃 DAY 2 Start day two by hiking north on the Bluff Trail beyond Big Devils Stairs Trail. The Bluff Trail remains mostly level, but it is very rocky, slowing your travel. Notice how the Bluff Trail's tread narrows beyond the Big Devils Stairs Trail as occasional, wide, shallow streambeds cross the trail. At mile 4.7, the trail begins an extended downhill, dropping 200 feet in 0.2 miles. Begin looking for large tulip trees and oak trees in the vicinity. Pass between some cabin-sized boulders at mile 5.2, then descend again to reach the intersection with the Mount Marshall Trail at mile 5.8. This hike continues left, following the Mount Marshall Trail north, but some additional exploration possibilities open up to the right. The Jordan River Trail, just 0.4 miles from this intersection, has several old homesites at the lower end of trail.

Continue north, stepping over Falls Branch at mile 5.9, then make a mild but steady ascent. Look for more big trees in the trailside woods. Enter a mountain laurel thicket on a rib ridge at mile 7. The canopy gives way overhead. Shortly reenter hardwoods and reach Sprucepine Branch at mile 7.2. It is broken into two branches. Beyond the second branch, begin to look for a campsite in the next mile or so. The land is steep near Sprucepine Branch, but levels enough for decent campsites between the branch and Waterfall Branch, 1 mile away.

🏃 DAY 3 Begin day three of your loop hike on the Mount Marshall Trail, as it curves around another laurel laden rib ridge beyond Sprucepine Branch. Before turning into the steep hollow of Waterfall Branch, resume passing through a hardwood forest, then camber past some level land with a vast number of downed tree trunks. Cross Waterfall Branch at mile 8.1. Climb away from the creek, working

around a ridge dividing Bolton Branch from
Waterfall Branch. Spindly striped maples line the
path. Level out and, before you know it, reach
Skyline Drive at mile 9.3. Turn right, walking down
alongside the parkway while wishing there were a
direct trail connection to the AT. Compton Peak is
dead ahead as you walk. Walk past Jenkins Gap
Overlook on your right, and at mile 9.6, turn left
into the Jenkins Gap parking area after crossing
Skyline Drive. Pick up the yellow-blazed Jenkins Gap
Trail and walk 150 feet to meet the AT. Turn left
(southbound) onto the AT.

Begin ascending an unnamed knob, crossing a
wide old roadbed. Pass three consecutive national
park survey markers before curving around a flat at
mile 10.2. Apple trees, relics of a pre-park orchard,
survive in the surrounding woods. Their fruits litter
the trail in September and October. Top out at mile
10.5, and then work downhill among broken woods
and sporadic clearings. Pass a small building foundation before reaching Skyline Drive at mile 11.2.
Cross Skyline Drive and begin the most continuous
climb of the hike. The grade is gentle at first, as it
traverses Hogwallow Flats in a hickory-oak woodland,
with sweet birch and striped maple as understory
trees. If you are thirsty, look for the short side trail
leading left to Hogwallow Flat Spring at mile 11.8.
The path is not signed, but rocks line it. The spring
is rocked in at the top with a pipe at its lower end.

Keep uphill, as the AT climbs in fits and starts,
generally ascending moderately in thick woods and
more sharply over bouldery locales. At mile 12.7, top
out on North Mount Marshall (elevation 3,368
feet). Here, mountain ash grows among the rocks. A
side trail leads right to a view, but an easier-to-reach
rock vista is just down-trail. More side trails lie
ahead. Soon, the AT opens directly to the edge of a
precipice. South Mount Marshall is visible in the
foreground, as is Hogback Mountain. Leave the vista
and make a rocky, slow descent back into canopied
woods, reaching the parking area at mile 13.3, ending your overnight trip.

DIRECTIONS: From Front Royal, drive south on Skyline
Drive for 15.9 miles to a parking area on the east side of
Skyline Drive, milepost 15.9, between Browntown Valley
Overlook and Range View Overlook.

Thornton River

TRAVEL THE ONCE-POPULATED *Thornton Hollow to camp along Thornton River and take a walk through history. Explore the midlands along Hull School Trail to Bolen Cemetery and hike up Keyser Run Fire Road into the high country. Camp along the headwaters of the Piney River and complete your loop on a pleasant stretch of the Appalachian Trail (AT). The hiking is neither long nor hard. Trout anglers and history buffs will especially enjoy this backpacking adventure.*

🥾 DAY 1 Start your hike from the Thornton River Trail parking area by descending through an open, oak and hickory forest on the Thornton River Trail. Begin paralleling a branch of the Thornton into the hollow. At mile 1.4 make your first crossing of the North Fork of the Thornton River. This river has a highly variable water flow, but it should be fairly easy to cross, except after a storm. It is also one of Shenandoah's more productive brook-trout streams.

Continue down Thornton Hollow and cross the river at mile 2.4. Soon, the trail makes a sharp right in an open area to cross the river at mile 2.7. Here, where the valley is wide, the imprint of man is visible on both sides of the river. Look for roads, rock walls, and rusty artifacts. Remember, these are cultural resources of the park and should be left where they are for others to enjoy. Cross the river again at mile 3, passing through an overgrown field to intersect the Hull School Trail at mile 3.1. The Hull School once stood to your right as you face downriver.

Continue forward on Thornton River Trail through a flat area covered with pines. Your first night's destination, there are many inviting spots from which to choose a campsite along Thornton River Trail.

🥾 DAY 2 Start Start day two by returning to Hull School Trail, turn right, and climb along a small stream. Step over the stream and wind your way 0.8 miles to a gap between Fork Mountain and Piney Ridge. You are now at mile 4.8 of your loop hike. Continue on Hull School Trail. On your way down, look for the straight gray trunks of the many tulip trees on the mountainside.

At mile 5.3, Hull School Trail and Piney Branch Trail coincide for 0.2 miles. Turn left and immediately cross Piney River. The Piney River valley was once heavily settled, too. At the next junction Hull School Trail splits off to the right. Follow it up and out of the Piney River valley to intersect Keyser Run Fire Road at mile 6.3.

Leave Hull School Trail and turn left on Keyser Run Fire Road. Immediately on your right is Bolen Cemetery. Red maples line the rock-walled pioneer burial plot. Continue climbing gently through piney woods, coming to a prolonged level stretch 0.6 miles past the cemetery. The ascent resumes, reaching a grassy clearing beneath a large red oak, before intersecting Pole Bridge Link Trail. At mile 8.7, come to the trail junction known as Fourway and make a sharp left on Pole Bridge Link Trail. Gently descend on the old road for 0.5 miles and reach the Sugarloaf Trail. Stay to the left on Pole Bridge Link Trail and begin to look for a campsite in the next mile or two. This is your second night's destination.

There are good campsites all around the area. Your water source is the upper reaches of the Piney River. To get water, head 0.4 miles farther on Pole Bridge Link Trail to Piney Branch Trail. Turn right on Piney Branch Trail and cross Piney River. You can get water here and return to your campsite.

🚶 DAY 3   Start by continuing down Pole Bridge Link Trail to Piney Branch Trail. Turn right on Piney Branch Trail, crossing the upper reaches of Piney River en route to the AT 1.3 miles ahead. Make a few very gentle and very wide switchbacks through an open forest with a grassy understory before coming to the AT at mile 10.9 of your loop hike.

Turn left on the AT and make southbound tracks, crossing a grassy lane before coming to the Range View Cabin service road. Follow it a short distance and veer left on the AT as it splits off again. Before intersecting the service road again at mile 11.4, pass a side trail (left) leading to the cabin. Cross the road at an angle and stay on the AT

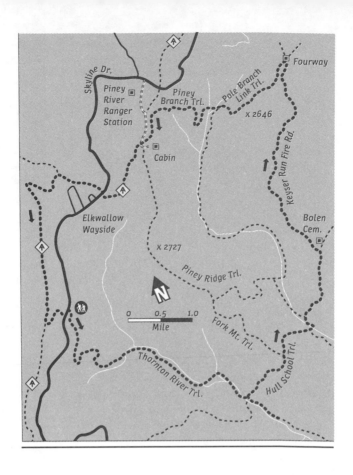

through open woods, making a 0.5-mile descent to
Skyline Drive. Cross Skyline Drive and veer right,
intersecting the Elkwallow Trail at mile 12.3. Stay on
the AT and make a sharp descent amid a picturesque
woodland carpeted in grass during the summer. As
the trail levels, you will pass the side trail to Elkwallow Picnic Area. Resume the downgrade, passing a
marked spring on your left before intersecting
Jeremys Run Trail at mile 12.9. Make a sharp left,
staying on the AT.

The AT crosses the spring branch and begins an
extended climb. Views of Knob Mountain open up
to your right. Round the point of a ridge at mile
13.4 but continue ascending along the top of the
ridge for another 0.5 miles. The forest has
encroached on both sides, but is open overhead.

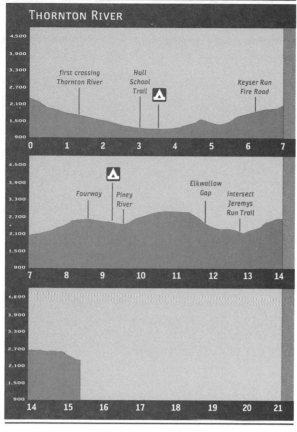

The trail keeps a level course as the ridge widens on one of the most pleasant stretches of the entire AT. Here the forest opens up again, offering obscured views of the ridge on either side. The easy hiking continues to the junction with Thornton River Trail at mile 15.

Turn left on the Thornton River Trail and descend through a ragged forest recovering from gypsy-moth damage. Make a sharp switchback to your right just before reaching Skyline Drive, completing your loop at mile 15.4. The Thornton River Trail parking area is a short distance to your left.

DIRECTIONS: From Thornton Gap, take Skyline Drive north for 9.4 miles to the Thornton River Trail parking area (on your right at milepost 25.4). It is 1 mile past the Jeremys Run Overlook. The Thornton River Trail starts on the left side of the parking area.

Neighbor Mountain/
Jeremys Run

SCENERY: ☆ ☆ ☆ ☆
DIFFICULTY: ☆ ☆
TRAIL CONDITION: ☆ ☆ ☆
SOLITUDE: ☆ ☆ ☆
CHILDREN: ☆ ☆ ☆
DISTANCE: *Day 1, 5.2 miles; Day 2, 5.2miles; Day 3, 4.4 miles*
HIKING TIME: *3:30, 3:45, and 3:00 hours*
OUTSTANDING *Features: views from the Neighbor, quality trout stream*

THIS OVERNIGHT LOOP PASSES OVER *the frequently-visited
Neighbor Mountain and down to Jeremys Run, one of the prettiest
and most productive trout streams in the park. Camp on the lower
reaches of this stream and make your way up to camp on nearby
Knob Mountain. Complete your loop on one of the most pleasant
stretches of the entire Appalachian Trail (AT). Busy weekends may
have a few other backpackers on the AT or Jeremys Run.*

🚶🚶 DAY 1 Start day one on a short spur trail
veering to the right from the southwest corner of the
Neighbor Mountain parking area. (Note: *Do not take
Neighbor Mountain Horse Trail.*) Take this spur trail 50
yards to intersect the AT. Turn left on the AT and
begin a winding climb up the western side of
Neighbor Mountain.

At 0.4 miles turn right on the Neighbor
Mountain Trail and trace a grassy path through a
thick woodland that hosts a dense understory of
mountain laurel and smaller trees. The trail then
heads westward, alternating between level and
descending stretches.

The woods become more attractive and open
with oaks above and grass below. At mile 1, make a
short ascent on an unnamed rocky knob.
Intermittent views open up on both sides as the ridge
narrows. Jeremys Run is below and to your right.
Knob Mountain is beyond it.

Hike over a second knob and reach a conspicu-
ous rock outcrop on your right at mile 1.4. Several
dark rocks stand upright amid smaller rounded
boulders. Hop up on a boulder and look over the
Shenandoah Valley, which spreads out to your right,
and the mountains of the park's Central District,
which hover on the skyline to your left.

Continue heading west on Neighbor Mountain,
passing bare trunks of gypsy moth—destroyed trees.

Enter a dense forest as you climb to the peak of The Neighbor at mile 2.4. The Potomac Appalachian Trail Club map states The Neighbor's peak elevation to be 2,725 feet.

Leave the mountain crest and descend down the steep north slope of The Neighbor. The foot-pounding drop ends at mile 5.1 as you intersect the Jeremys Run Trail, just after passing a fern field. To continue on your loop hike, turn right onto Jeremys Run Trail, but you will want to begin searching for suitable campsites for your first night's destination. These can be found a mile upstream or downstream along Jeremys Run from this turning point. While here, you can explore Jeremys Run west to its exit from park boundaries. Also, good fishing and swimming holes are nearby with big rocks to sun on.

🚶🚶 DAY 2   Begin by heading up Jeremys Run Trail on a mild grade, passing a small cascade on your right at mile 5.8. Rock walls line the path through here, and white pines grow on former fields along the trail. Sycamores shade the stream where brook trout gather in deep pools.

Where rock bluffs crowd the stream, the trail crosses to the other side toward flatter terrain. This pattern of crowding and crossing continues up the valley. In times of high water these fords will become dangerous, but most of the time you can cross the run dry-shod.

At mile 8.9 the trail appears to end on a mud bluff overlooking the creek. Here the trail has been washed out from a flood. Continue carefully along the bluff and pick up the path again in 40 feet. More crossings and a steadier grade bring you to the head of the valley and the junction with Knob Mountain Cutoff Trail at mile 9.9. Turn left on Knob Mountain Cutoff Trail and cross Jeremys Run one last time. Get your water here for use at the forth-coming night's camp. There is no water along the crest of Knob Mountain.

Wind your way to the crest of Knob Mountain, about a half-mile walk. You can find campsites in either direction from here along Knob Mountain Trail. This is your second night's destination.

🚶🚶 DAY 3   Start day three by dropping back to Jeremys Run on Knob Mountain Cutoff Trail. Turn left on Jeremys Run Trail and ascend to the AT at mile 11.4 of your loop hike. Then make a right, heading southbound on the AT.

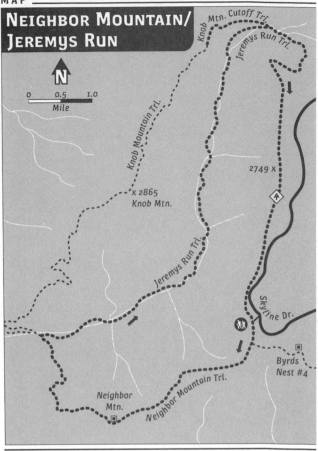

NEIGHBOR MOUNTAIN/ JEREMYS RUN

Knob Mtn. Cutoff Trl.

Jeremys Run Trl.

Knob Mountain Trl.

2749 x

x 2865
Knob Mtn.

Jeremys Run Trl.

Skyline Dr.

Byrds
Nest #4

Neighbor
Mtn.

Neighbor Mountain Trl.

0   0.5   1.0
Mile

   The AT crosses a spring branch and begins an
extended climb with views of Knob Mountain opening up to your right. Round the point of a ridge at
mile 11.9 but continue ascending along the top of
the ridge for another 0.5 miles. The forest has
encroached on both sides but is open overhead.
   The trail keeps a level course as the ridge widens
on one of the most pleasant stretches of the entire
AT. Here the forest canopy opens again, offering
obscured views of the ridge on either side. The easy
hiking continues to the junction with Thornton
River Trail at mile 13.5.
   The path makes a mild downgrade, parallels
Skyline Drive, and passes just below the Jeremys Run
Overlook. You'll soon come to the spur trail leading
to The Neighbor Mountain parking area at mile 14.7.
Turn left on the spur trail and complete your loop.

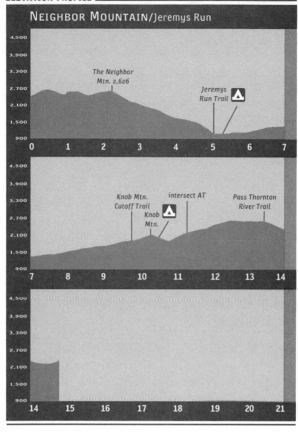

NEIGHBOR MOUNTAIN/Jeremys Run

DIRECTIONS: From Thornton Gap, take Skyline Drive north for 4.7 miles to the Neighbor Mountain parking area at milepost 26.8. The unmarked parking area will be 0.8 miles past the Thornton Hollow Overlook on the left side of Skyline Drive. The hike starts in the southwest corner of the parking area.

Hazel Country

SCENERY: ✿ ✿ ✿ ✿

DIFFICULTY: ✿ ✿ ✿

TRAIL CONDITION: ✿ ✿ ✿

SOLITUDE: ✿ ✿ ✿

CHILDREN: ✿ ✿ ✿

DISTANCE: DAY 1, *4.2 miles; Day 2, 7 miles; Day 3, 6.6 miles*

HIKING TIME: *3:00, 5:15, and 5:00 hours*

OUTSTANDING FEATURES: *multiple homesites, waterfall, views, rock "cave"*

THIS OVERNIGHT LOOP MEANDERS THROUGH *"Hazel Country,"*
one of the most heavily settled areas prior to the establishment of the
park. Head down the Hazel River, pass by a waterfall and rock
"cave," and camp on the lower reaches of the river. Return to more
lofty terrain on the steep Sams Ridge Trail and then traverse a series
of flat-topped mountains into Nicholson Hollow. Pitch your tent
where fields and farms once stood. Complete your loop by hiking
along Hannah Run with its many artifacts from pioneer days. This is
the most history-laden loop in this book.

🚶 DAY 1 Leave Skyline Drive on the Hazel
Mountain Trail from the Spring Mountain parking
area and come to a trail junction at 0.5 miles. Veer
right on the Hazel Mountain Trail, which tunnels
through a forest with dense canopy overhead. Soon
the trail bears left, levels out, and crosses several
small springs draining off Buck Ridge to the left.

The trail sidles Hazel River at 1 mile, then continues along the river and intersects White Rocks
Trail at mile 1.6. Turn left on White Rocks Trail. As
the trail ascends slightly and then levels out along an
old road, the forest changes from moisture-tolerant
hardwoods, such as maple, to pine and chestnut oak
as it crests the ridgetop.

The trail becomes rockier and descends somewhat, coming to an unmarked junction at mile 2.3.
The main trail continues forward, while a footpath
turns right. Follow the unmarked footpath down an
eroded, rocky, and steep path.

Reach the river in 0.2 mile. Turn right, following the footpath 0.5 mile upstream to a waterfall.
On your right a rock indentation lies at the base of a
huge granite bluff. Nearby, a waterfall drops about
30 feet down a narrow chute into a deep pool.

Return to White Rocks Trail and turn right. The
trail continues to descend, angling the left side of the

ridge. Look for a rock outcrop to the left at mile 2.6, where you have a pine-framed view of Skyline Drive, Buck Ridge, and the backside of Marys Rock. The trail is varied in character according to its level of exposure. Where it is moist, tulip trees and northern red oak thrive; in drier areas, pine and mountain laurel dominate. Watch for another outcrop to your left that's a great spot to catch some views to the east.

Next, the trail steeply descends to a gap at mile 3.7. Notice the triple-trunked oak tree here. Veer to the right and head down 0.2 miles to Hazel River. Cross the river and pass through a flat area, stepping over a small creek that enters from your right. Intersect and turn left onto the Hazel River Trail at mile 4. Head downstream and begin to look for a campsite in the next mile or so. This is your first night's destination.

🏃 DAY 2 Start day two by continuing down the Hazel River Trail. As the hollow narrows, you'll cross the river for the first of four times within 0.7 miles. The trail then nears the stream before arriving at Sams Ridge Trail at mile 5.6. Turn right on Sams Ridge Trail and immediately begin climbing, leaving the park confines. Pass an abandoned shack on your right as the trail rounds the east slope of Sams Ridge. Reenter the park at mile 6.2 and look for sizeable oak trees.

The steep grade levels out briefly by a rock wall but resumes climbing up to mile 7.2, where you'll arrive at an old homesite on the left. After crossing a spring, the walking is easy to Broad Hollow Trail at mile 7.6. Turn right at the junction. Both trails share the same path to Hazel Mountain Trail at mile 7.8. Turn left on the Hazel Mountain Trail, which heads 0.5 miles through crowded woods to another trail junction. Continue forward through the junction, staying in pine woodland on the Hazel Mountain Trail.

An obscure trail comes in from your left at mile 8.8. Veer right, picking up the Hot—Short Mountain Trail, which skirts the south side of Catlett Mountain. Intermittent views of Old Rag open up to your left. Look for an old chimney on your left at mile 9.7 and drop down to cross a side stream. The trail then turns away from the creek and descends farther, heading through rock walls at mile 10.7. Intersect Nicholson Hollow Trail at mile 11.

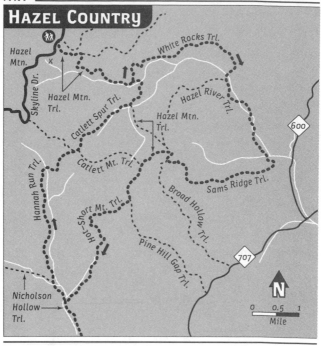

HAZEL COUNTRY

Turn left on the Nicholson Hollow Trail until the river comes into view. Begin to look for campsites within the next mile or so in the flat to your left. This is your second night's destination.

🥾 DAY 3 Begin your third day by heading back up the Nicholson Hollow Trail. Continue beyond the Hot–Short Mountain Trail and cross Hannah Run. Come to the Hannah Run Trail at mile 11.7. Veer right, traversing a flat with rock walls, rock piles, and a chimney on your left. Walk along Hannah Run as it descends through a hemlock forest.

Rock piles abound in this second-growth woodland. A rock wall and the creek hem you in at mile 12.3. The rocky trail veers away from Hannah Run and parallels the stream high above the run. Pass a mostly intact chimney and a few rusted-out washtubs marking an old homesite at mile 13.1. The roofless frame of an old cabin stands just to the left of the trail at mile 13.5. Descend to Hannah Run, step over the stream, and begin a very tough 0.2-mile climb out of the watershed. The walking is much easier for the remaining distance to a trail junction at mile 14.2.

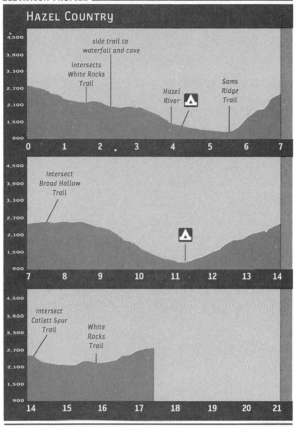

Veer right, going downhill on Catlett Mountain Trail for 0.1 mile and approach a second junction. Turn left on the Catlett Spur Trail and continue descending, as you drift off and on an old road among the headwaters of Runyons Run. Cross Runyons Runs at mile 14.9 and hike a nearly level course before coming to the Hazel Mountain Trail at mile 15.4. Turn left on Hazel Mountain Trail and traverse a small ridge before dropping to cross Hazel River. You will reach the junction with the White Rocks Trail at mile 16. Retrace your steps up the Hazel Mountain Trail to arrive at Skyline Drive completing your loop (mile 17.6).

DIRECTIONS: From Thornton Gap, take Skyline Drive south for 2 miles to the Meadow Spring parking area at milepost 33.5. The parking area is on the left side of Skyline Drive.

Hughes River

SCENERY: ✿ ✿ ✿ ✿ ✿

DIFFICULTY: ✿ ✿

TRAIL CONDITION: ✿ ✿ ✿

SOLITUDE: ✿ ✿

CHILDREN: ✿ ✿ ✿

DISTANCE: *Day 1, 4.4miles; Day 2, 5.7miles; Day 3, 2.3 miles*

HIKING TIME: *3:00, 4:15, and 1:30 hours*

OUTSTANDING FEATURES: *old homesites, great views, cabin ruins*

THIS LOOP STARTS IN THE EASTERN lowlands of Shenandoah and heads up Hughes River, once heavily settled by mountain folk. It then heads deep into the hills, passing over Robertson Mountain with its wonderful views. Next, drop down to camp in Brokenback Run before leaving the park. Backpackers may want to include a layover day at Brokenback Run for a side hike up to Old Rag. The angling is good on Hughes River.

🚶 DAY 1 Leave the Old Rag parking area and head up VA 600 for 0.5 miles to Nicholson Hollow Trail, which starts on your right. Trace the gravel road and bear right at a sign for the trail. Walk 50 rocky yards to cross Brokenback Run and Hughes River in succession. You may have to wade here. The wide trail hugs the right bank of Hughes River and reaches the park boundary at 0.8 miles.

Pass former farmland as the trail moves away from the river. At mile 1.2 a side path leads left to a large pool in Hughes River, a potential swimming hole during warmer months. The trail enters an area of huge boulders and emerges riverside at mile 1.5. The Corbin Mountain Trail comes in from across the river, but stay on the Nicholson Hollow Trail, passing through more farmland.

Intersect the Hot-Short Mountain Trail at mile 1.9. Continue forward, cross Hannah Run, and traverse the spit of land between Hughes River and Hannah Run. Pass the Hannah Run Trail at mile 2.2. After crossing Hughes River at mile 2.7, the path steepens beneath a diminishing hemlock wood. Climb away from the river but come to the river again at mile 3.9, the site of a former settlement. Begin to look for potential campsites within the next mile or two. Soon you will come to a sign tacked on a sweet birch indicating a spring. The fields to your left are growing up. At mile 4.3, just beyond the sign and brushy fields to your left, is a crumbling chimney, a rocky streambed, the Corbin Cabin, and a trail junction

More potential campsites lie across the Hughes River on the Corbin Cabin Cutoff Trail. Walk a short distance up this trail—notice cabin ruins to your left. From here, walk directly downstream a couple of hundred yards to a white-pine grove with many rock walls. This general area is your first night's destination. Trail etiquette requires that you camp out of sight of the trail.

🚶 DAY 2 Start Start day two by continuing on or returning to the Nicholson Hollow Trail. Head uptrail and cross the often-dry Indian Run streambed before arriving at a trail junction at mile 4.7. Turn left on the Indian Run Trail, which ascends a rock-lined woods road. The trail veers left at mile 4.9 and steepens as you step over stone waterbars, which keep the trail from eroding. Cove hardwoods dominate the forest: birch, basswood, and sugar maple. Cross several often-dry streambeds emanating from the slopes of Stony Man Mountain. The trail begins to level out in fern-floored woods and actually descends a bit before nearing a junction at mile 6.3.

Turn right on the Corbin Mountain Trail and swing around the headwaters of Brokenback Run. Climb gently and come to the wide-open Old Rag Fire Road at mile 6.9. Turn left on Old Rag Fire Road. Pass the Corbin Hollow Trail at mile 7.4 and begin looking for the Robertson Mountain Trail just ahead on which you should turn left. The footpath enters a laurel thicket, turns back to the right, and switchbacks up among rocks and trees. At mile 8.3 the trail passes by the summit of Robertson Mountain on your right. Look for a spur trail on the right that leads to various outcrops and cleared overlooks along Skyline Drive. The hump of Hawksbill looms tall in the southwest.

Leave the top of Robertson Mountain toward Brokenback Run, but not before getting an obscured view of Old Rag from an outcrop on your left. The rigorous descent proceeds toward Brokenback Run without the benefit of many switchbacks. This thigh-burning descent levels off a mile from the top in an open area that hosts more views of Old Rag. Start downward again, entering the moist valley of Brokenback Run. Follow the run and come to Weakley Hollow Fire Road, 1.6 miles from the summit of Robertson Mountain. Turn left on the fire road

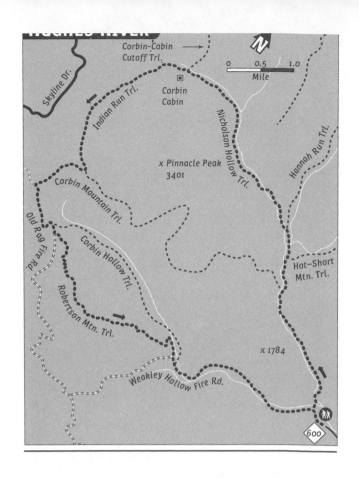

Corbin-Cabin
Cutoff Trl.

Skyline Dr.

Indian Run Trl.

Corbin
Cabin

Nicholson Hollow Trl.

Hannah Run Trl.

x Pinnacle Peak
3401

Corbin Mountain Trl.

Old Rag Fire Rd.

Corbin Hollow Trl.

Robertson Mtn. Trl.

Hot–Short
Mtn. Trl.

x 1784

Weakley Hollow Fire Rd.

600

0   0.5   1.0
Mile

ELEVATION PROFILE

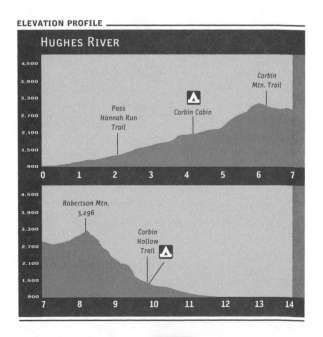

HUGHES RIVER

4,500
3,900
3,300
2,700
2,100
1,500
900

Pass
Hannah Run
Trail

Corbin Cabin

Corbin
Mtn. Trail

0   1   2   3   4   5   6   7

4,500
3,900
3,300
2,700
2,100
1,500
900

Robertson Mtn.
3,296

Corbin
Hollow
Trail

7   8   9   10   11   12   13   14

and intersect Corbin Hollow Trail at mile 10. Turn left and head upstream, crossing the run. Begin to look for a campsite in the next couple of miles. This is your second night's destination. This camp makes a great base camp for a side trip to Old Rag.

🏃 DAY 3   Begin day three by returning to Weakley Hollow Fire Road. Turn left and cross Brokenback Run on a metal bridge. As you walk the road, look for the large, 18- to 24-inch leaves of the umbrella magnolia tree. The unmistakable leaves are pointed at both ends. The umbrella magnolia prefers low-elevation, streamside environments.

Cross Brokenback Run again on three foot-bridges and then span a side stream on yet another footbridge, coming to a parking area at mile 11.7. Walk down VA 600 for 0.8 miles to the Old Rag parking area, completing your loop at mile 12.5.

DIRECTIONS: From Thornton Gap on Skyline Drive, drive east on US 211 for 6.5 miles to US 522 in Sperryville. Turn right, heading southeast, and follow US 522 for 0.5 miles to VA 231. Turn right on VA 231 and head south for 7 miles to VA 601 (Peola Mills Road). There is a sign for Old Rag Mountain. Turn right on VA 601 and drive 0.3 miles to VA 600 (Nethers Road) and turn right. Stay on the main road, passing through the small community of Nethers, and arrive at the Old Rag parking area on your left after 2.6 miles. Start your loop here.

Jones Mountain

SCENERY: ✪ ✪ ✪ ✪ ✪
DIFFICULTY: ✪ ✪
TRAIL CONDITION: ✪ ✪ ✪
SOLITUDE: ✪ ✪ ✪ ✪
CHILDREN: ✪ ✪ ✪
DISTANCE: *Day 1, 6.6 miles; Day 2, 5.4 miles; Day 3, 1.8 miles*
HIKING TIME: *5:00, 5:00, and 2:00 hours*
OUTSTANDING FEATURES: *good views, good fishing, scenic valleys, solitude*

THIS LOOP IS CHOCK-FULL OF PICTURESQUE *highs and equally scenic lows. Enjoy rolling, ridgetop walking along Jones Mountain to a great view at Bear Church Rock. Then drop down and camp along the pretty Staunton River valley near a former homesite. Enjoy more of the river valley as you head up the Staunton and then drop down*

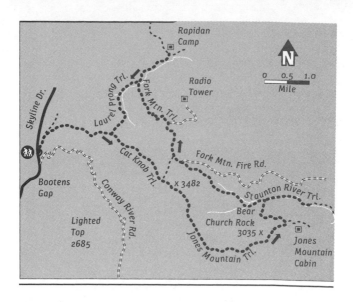

to the Laurel Prong valley and camp there. A worthwhile side trip to
Rapidan Camp is not more than a mile away. Complete your loop by
returning to the high country and Bootens Gap. This is one of the
best overnight loops in the Central District.

🚶 DAY 1 Head north on the Appalachian Trail
(AT) from the rear of the Bootens Gap parking area.
The AT moderately ascends the southwest side of
Hazeltop. At a trail junction at 0.4 miles, turn right
on the Laurel Prong Trail to descend past several
springs on a boulder-laden slope. The trail drops
sharply just before arriving at breezy Laurel Gap and
another trail junction at mile 1.4.

Continue forward, now on the Cat Knob Trail,
which winds uphill, twisting and turning among gray
boulders. Veer right on the Jones Mountain Trail at
mile 2.1, skirting the Rapidan Wildlife Management
Area.

This ridge-running trail makes for pleasant
walking among windswept oaks. The fern and grass
understory, mingled with mountain laurel, makes
the path even more appealing. The little-used trail
descends, making an unexpected right turn at mile
2.6. Pass through a gap in a broken forest and reenter the park at mile 2.9 in an oak woodland. Begin
an extensive level stretch that slopes slightly downhill.

In a grassy gap at mile 3.5, the trail turns left and
downward, heading east toward Bear Church Rock
and away from Bluff Mountain. Look for an outcrop

ELEVATION PROFILE _____

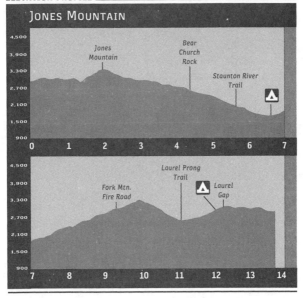

on your left with views of Fork Mountain and then begin a roller-coaster descent along Jones Mountain among large granite outcrops in the woods.

The trail zigzags very steeply down the crest of the ridge between brush and laurel at mile 4.4. Watch for a side trail splitting to the left in 0.1 mile; it emerges onto the granite slab of Bear Church Rock, which makes for a natural viewing platform. Fork Mountain, Doubletop Mountain, and the crest of the Blue Ridge stand out. Below you is the Staunton River.

Return to the main trail and switchback precipitously, coming to a junction at mile 5. The locked Jones Mountain Cabin is to your right. Turn left on a milder grade, passing through a tunnel of mountain laurel before intersecting the McDaniel Hollow Trail at mile 5.3. Veer right, still descending on a spur ridge, and find the Staunton River Trail at mile 5.7.

Turn right, heading down the Staunton River Trail, and immediately pass an eroded wash. Former homesites occupy the flats to your right. The trail comes alongside the creek at mile 6.5, where the riverbed shows the effects of the flood of 1995. Look for stone walls and rock piles at mile 6.6. Begin to scope out a campsite in the next mile or two along the Staunton River. This is your first night's destination.

🏃 DAY 2 Start day two by returning up the Staunton River Trail for 0.9 miles to the Jones

Mountain Trail. Parallel the Staunton River, which is far below you. Although you will notice many stumps, the attractive woods are heavy with birch. Intersect the McDaniel Hollow Trail coming in from your left at mile 8 and immediately cross a small stream coming from the hollow. On your left you will see a huge pile of chestnut boards at an old homesite.

Pass the branches of Garth Spring Run. Drop down and cross the river at 8.2 miles. You will see another pile of chestnut boards on your right before you again step over the pretty watercourse with its small falls and pools. The footpath becomes irregular and steep, crowding close to the stream before turning sharply left at the falls of mile 8.6. Enter a hemlock forest fighting for survival and reach Fork Mountain Fire Road at mile 9.4.

Head left up the fire road as it easily winds along the head of the valley to a trail junction at mile 10.1. Many hemlocks have succumbed to the woolly adelgid here. Be sure to take the Fork Mountain Trail, which leads downhill, not the Jones Mountain Trail, which makes an acute left.

The Fork Mountain Trail follows a rocky, eroded course as it switchbacks down toward Laurel Prong. Striped maples grow in abundance along the upper trail and two giant oak trees stand guard over the trail as it switchbacks at mile 10.6. Soon the switchbacks end and the path heads straight down into a wide and picturesque fern field. It reaches Laurel Prong at mile 11.2. The stream is sluggish here and makes for a potentially muddy crossing. The trail tends downstream but climbs up and away from Laurel Prong, intersecting the Laurel Prong Trail at 11.3.

Turn left on the Laurel Prong Trail, passing evidence of old homesites, including a chimney at mile 11.8. Then cross a small stream, climb a hill, and begin to look for campsites on either side of the trail in the next mile or so. This is your second night's destination. A side trip back down to Rapidan Camp is worth the 1-mile hike. There, you can explore the mountain getaway of former president Herbert Hoover.

🐾 DAY 3   Start day three by continuing up Laurel Prong Trail, which begins to climb more steeply. Mountain laurel appears trailside before you reach Laurel Gap in a deep, dark forest at mile 12.4. Turn right, staying on the Laurel Prong Trail, retracing your steps, and coming to the AT at mile 13.4.

Turn left on the AT, heading south downhill. Return
to Bootens Gap at mile 13.8, completing your loop.

DIRECTIONS: From Swift Run Gap, head north on Skyline
Drive for 10.4 miles to the Bootens Gap parking area (mile
55.3). The small parking area is on your right. The
Appalachian Trail starts in the back of the parking area.

Conway River

SCENERY: ☆ ☆ ☆ ☆
DIFFICULTY: ☆ ☆
TRAIL CONDITION: ☆ ☆ ☆ ☆
SOLITUDE: ☆ ☆ ☆
CHILDREN: ☆ ☆ ☆
DISTANCE: Day 1, 4.6 miles; Day 2, 3.8 miles; Day 3, 3.6 miles
HIKING TIME: 3:30, 3:45, and 3:00 hours
OUTSTANDING FEATURES: good campsites, great views, a rock scramble, old trees

THIS LOOP LEAVES THE BLUE RIDGE *and follows the scenic
Conway River through part of the Rapidan Wildlife Management
Area. Leave the Conway River and head into the high country on the
rarely trampled Slaughter Trail, passing a pioneer homesite, to camp
on the upper reaches of Devils Ditch. Complete your trip by clam-
bering over Bearfence Mountain, with its 360-degree views, on a
short but challenging rock scramble. The daily mileages are low,
making this a good break-in trip for novice backpackers.*

🚶 DAY 1 Leave the Bootens Gap parking area
on Conway River Fire Road and make two switchbacks on the way to the river. Come to the upper
Conway River, which may be dry here at 0.7 miles.
Swing away from the watercourse then pass through a
gate at 1.4 miles. Enter the Rapidan Wildlife
Management Area. Red blazes mark the boundary
between the national park and the wildlife area.

Swing back left and cross an often-dry ravine at
mile 1.6. Over the next couple of miles you may see a
4WD vehicle on the road. Rough 4WD roads splinter
off the main path. Cross a fair-sized stream at mile
2.6 and then arrive at a fork in the road. The left fork
leads to a large clearing. Stay on the right fork leading
to Bootens Run. Cross the stream and come alongside
the boulder-strewn Conway River at mile 3.3. The
national park is on the far side of the stream.

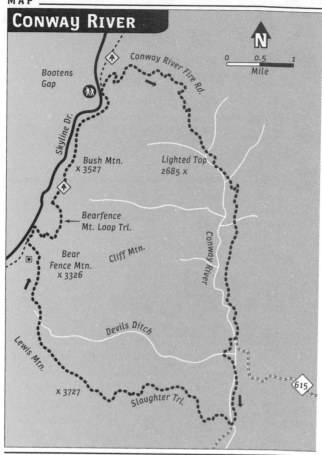

Stay left at the next fork in the road. Pass a small creek and campsite to your left at mile 4. Keep descending and come to yet another fork and VA 615 (mile 4.2). A sign reads, "End of State Maintenance." Make a hairpin turn to the right and start down to Conway River. It looks like the trail ends on a bluff at the river, but the rest of the trail bed has been washed away. Make your way carefully across the river, leaving any potential jeep traffic behind. Head slightly upstream and reach a washed out roadbed.

Turn left, heading down Conway River, which is now on your left. Keep your eyes peeled for a campsite in the next mile or so. You will pass along the densely forested river and cross Devils Ditch at mile 4.6. This is your first night's destination.

🥾 DAY 2 Start day two by returning to the main trail and following the Conway River downstream.

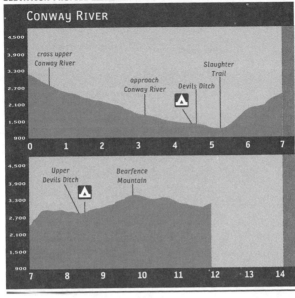

Pass a side trail that leads to Devils Ditch and soon cross Conway River at mile 4.9 . Evidence of flood damage can be seen along the river—piled tree trunks, scoured roots, and jumbled rocks. The trail leads uphill, descends to the river, and forks at mile 5.3. The right fork leads to the river. Look across the deep pool in the river for the Slaughter Trail's concrete marker. This pool is a great summertime swimming hole. Cross the river here; this could be a wet ford.

Come to the marker for Slaughter Trail and begin heading upstream. Do not take the jeep road heading downstream along the river. Conway River should now be on your right. The rocky Slaughter Trail briefly parallels the watercourse then turns away to the left and begins climbing steeply up a spur ridge leading toward Lewis Mountain. Notice the old-growth white pines above you. The hemlocks have died.

The path switchbacks left at mile 5.7 and then steepens even more before leveling off at mile 6.3. Congratulations, you have just climbed 800 feet in 1 mile. Traverse a gap, pass a rock pile, climb a little more, then come to a homesite on your right. The chimney and foundation are crumbling. A spring is on the far side of the homesite.

Keep ascending on the eroded trail, passing blazed boundary trees. Pass the ruins of an outbuilding on your left and a split-rail fence on your right. At mile 7 beneath a yellow birch is a rock-lined spring sending forth cool water. The moss-covered trail nears Lewis Mountain, levels out at mile 7.5, and then cruises along the east slope of the mountain. But this little-maintained and rarely hiked trail is liable to have a few fallen trees along its course.

Over the next mile or two begin to look for a campsite. Meanwhile, start an irregular descent toward the upper Devils Ditch at mile 7.9, coming to the stream in 0.5 miles. The valley of upper Devils Ditch is your second night's destination. This is a short day, distance-wise, but the climb on the Slaughter Trail is tough in spots.

🚶 DAY 3   Start day three by continuing along the Slaughter Trail. The grassy trail is easy on your feet and lungs. Parallel a Devils Ditch feeder stream to a road fork. Keep going forward and reach the Appalachian Trail (AT) at mile 9.3. Turn right on the AT, heading north.

Ascend the AT and make a sharp right in a pine stand at mile 9.5. You are now on the southwest side of Bearfence Mountain. Switchback uphill among lichen-covered boulders, passing a rock on your right that has views of Bluff Mountain. Come to Bearfence Mountain Loop Trail at mile 9.8. Turn right, taking the loop trail, and keep climbing. A short trail leads left to the obscure crest of Bearfence Mountain. Descend a bit and pass an outcrop on your left with views of Skyline Drive, Massanutten Mountain, and the Shenandoah Valley.

Come to the Bearfence Mountain rock scramble and turn right. The scramble is doable with a backpack. Carefully follow the blue blazes and some fantastic views will open up in all directions, including the Conway River drainage from where you came. Return to the AT at mile 10.3 and turn right. The walk is easy, skirting the edge of Bush Mountain beneath some large oak trees. A prolonged descent nears Skyline Drive and then makes a final climb before coming to Conway River Fire Road at mile 12. Take a few steps left on the fire road and complete your loop at Bootens Gap.

DIRECTIONS: From Swift Run Gap, head north on Skyline Drive for 10.4 miles to the Bootens Gap parking area. The small parking area is on your right. Conway River Fire Road starts in the back of the parking area.

Rockytop/*Big Run*

> SCENERY: ☆ ☆ ☆ ☆ ☆
> DIFFICULTY: ☆ ☆
> TRAIL CONDITION: ☆ ☆ ☆
> SOLITUDE: ☆ ☆ ☆
> CHILDREN: ☆ ☆ ☆
> DISTANCE: *Day 1, 4.1miles; Day 2, 6.3 miles; Day 3, 4.8 miles*
> HIKING TIME: *3:00, 4:45,and 3:30*
> OUTSTANDING FEATURES: *Big Run watershed, views from Lewis Peak and Rockytop*

THIS LOOP FIRST TAKES YOU ALONG *high ridges to Lewis Mountain. Great views are just minutes from your first night's camp. Traverse Rockytop and catch more views before dropping into Big Run for some streamside camping in the park's largest watershed. Then climb out of Big Run back into the high country. Lewis Mountain should be all yours, whereas Big Run sees a few campers and fishermen. Be advised:* you must carry your water for your first night's camp.

🚶 DAY 1 Leave the Browns Gap parking area and easily descend on Madison Run Fire Road. The Browns Gap Turnpike, built in 1805, used this same route. Later, Civil War troops crossed the Blue Ridge here. At 0.8 miles, after a sharp right turn, look for a trail marker on your right. This is the Madison Run Spur Trail. Turn right and follow it 0.3 miles to a gap and another trail junction.

Turn left onto the Rockytop Trail, which undulates along a ridgetop and arrives at yet another trail junction at mile 1.6. Bear right, staying on the Rockytop Trail. The trail maintains a nearly level course, offering views of the Blue Ridge and Big Run. Gypsy moths have defoliated the trees that would ordinarily obscure this view.

Come to a sag at mile 2.2 and swing to the southwest of another knob. The vegetation changes to pine—mountain laurel woodland. Cross over a rock field, coming to another gap. The trail then straddles the ridge while passing over a couple of small knobs.

Turn left at a trail junction at mile 3.4, picking up the little-used Lewis Peak Trail. The trailside brush may be overgrown. The path descends steadily westward and confronts a scree slope on both sides of the ridge. Step out. To your left are the boulders of Blackrock and Furnace Mountain. To your right are views of Massanutten Mountain and Rockytop.

ROCKYTOP/BIG RUN

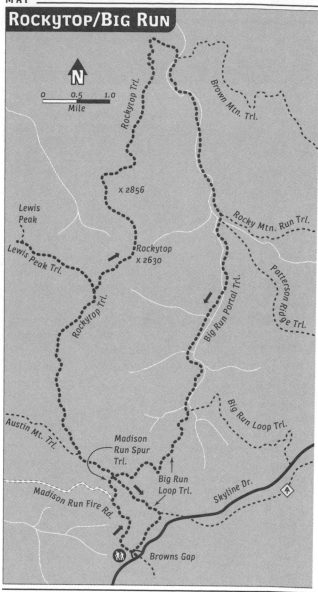

Lewis Peak

Lewis Peak Trl.

Rockytop Trl.

x 2856

Rockytop x 2630

Rockytop Trl.

Brown Mtn. Trl.

Rocky Mtn. Run Trl.

Patterson Ridge Trl.

Big Run Portal Trl.

Big Run Loop Trl.

Austin Mt. Trl.

Madison Run Spur Trl.

Big Run Loop Trl.

Skyline Dr.

Madison Run Fire Rd.

Browns Gap

0   0.5   1.0
Mile

N

Begin to look for a campsite along the ridgecrest for the next mile or so. This area is your first night's destination. Remember, there is no water up here. Continue to descend to a gap at 4.1 mile. The summit of Lewis Peak and its incredible views are just 0.3 miles away. Lewis Peak is also a great place to watch the sun rise over the Blue Ridge.

🚶 DAY 2 Start day two by returning to the Rockytop Trail. Turn left, begin descending, and pass the scree slope of Rockytop with good views into

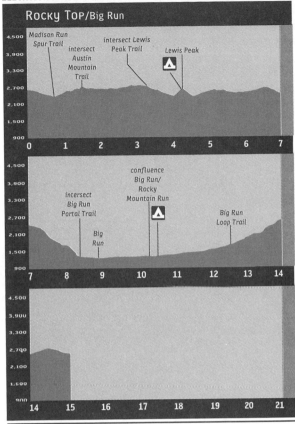

Rocky Top/Big Run

Big Run and the Shenandoah Valley. Drop again and, at mile 6.3, climb along the open slope of what many hikers refer to as the real Rockytop. With views of Lewis Peak to your south and the Shenandoah Valley beyond, this Rockytop offers better views than the first scree slope.

Top over an adjacent ridge of this peak and begin the sharp drop to Big Run. At mile 8.5, turn right onto the Big Run Portal Trail and head up along Big Run. Span Big Run on a wide, metal bridge and approach a trail junction at mile 9.

Stay on the old road that is Big Run Portal Trail and, at mile 9.2, rock hop Big Run. Leave a forest that is recovering from a 1986 fire and reach a second ford. This one can be crossed dry-shod at normal water levels but is more challenging than the first. Look for the long, blue-green needles and evenly spaced branches of white pines along the run.

Make easier crossings of Big Run in succession and reach a trail junction at mile 10.4. Big Run and Rocky Mountain Run come together here, forming a large and relatively flat drainage basin. This is your second night's destination. Look around; there are several suitable campsites a mile or more up each run. Explore the Big Run valley and look for evidence of old homesites.

🚶 DAY 3   Start day three by crossing Rocky Mountain Run and continuing on the Big Run Portal Trail. Intersect the Patterson Ridge Trail at mile 10.6 of your loop hike. Stay on the Big Run Portal Trail, fording Big Run and its feeder streams several times. At normal water levels, these should all be dry crossings.

Intersect the Big Run Loop Trail in an area where several feeder streams come together at mile 12.7. Take the fork to the right, climbing the steep trail along Big Run tributary. The Big Run Loop Trail switchbacks up to a gap and another trail junction at mile 14. Turn left, staying on the Big Run Loop Trail as it ascends gently. Cross an open knob before intersecting the Appalachian Trail (AT) at mile 14.6. Turn right on the AT and swing southward and down to complete your 15.2-mile loop at Browns Gap.

DIRECTIONS: From the Rockfish Gap entrance station take Skyline Drive north for 21.6 miles to Browns Gap parking area at milepost 83, which will be on your left.

Furnace Mountain/
Trayfoot Mountain

SCENERY: ☆ ☆ ☆ ☆ ☆
DIFFICULTY: ☆ ☆ ☆
TRAIL CONDITION: ☆ ☆ ☆ ☆
SOLITUDE: ☆ ☆ ☆
CHILDREN: ☆ ☆
DISTANCE: DAY 1, *6 miles; Day 2, 8.4 miles; Day 3, 6.2 miles*
HIKING TIME: *4:15, 6:30, and 4:45 hours*
OUTSTANDING FEATURES: *views from several peaks, Blackrock Springs*

IF YOU LIKE MOUNTAINTOP VIEWS AND CAMPING *along streams, this loop is for you. Head north on the Appalachian Trail (AT) and turn west toward Austin Mountain, with many views of* your destination. Camp in the woods along Madison Run and then climb up to Furnace Mountain for more views. Walk along the crest of Trayfoot Mountain and drop to Paine Run for more streamside camping. Pass historic Blackrock Springs and culminate your rewarding trip at the view from Blackrock.

🏃 DAY 1 Start your first day on the AT hiking northbound from the Jones Run parking area. Intermittent mountain views open up to your right. The AT descends gently to Browns Gap at mile 1.2. Cross Skyline Drive and continue north on the AT. Climb out of Browns Gap, reaching a trail junction at 1.8 miles, and then turn left onto Big Run Loop Trail. The grass-lined path ambles west and reaches another trail junction at mile 2.4.

Continue forward through the junction. You are now on the Rockytop Trail, which undulates along the ridgetop and arrives at the Austin Mountain Trail at mile 2.8. Bear left on the Austin Mountain Trail, making a westward track far below an unnamed knob. At mile 3.2, look left for views of Blackrock, a visible rock summit, and Trayfoot Mountain. Eventually, you'll be on top of both of these.

Soon the trail drops sharply down the spine of a ridge and continues through grassy woodland. Make a sharp switchback to the left and hit a gap at mile 4.1. Work your way along the south side of Austin Mountain and enjoy views of Shenandoah Valley and the mountains beyond while crossing a series of talus slopes.

At mile 5.5, make a sharp switchback to the left, where the trail begins to drop nearly 500 feet in the next 0.5 miles. Turn back to the right along a wet-weather draw and descend, intersecting Madison Run Fire Road at mile 6. Located 0.7 miles downstream and 1 mile upstream along Madison Run are many appealing streamside campsites. This will be your first night's destination.

🏃 DAY 2 Start day two by heading downstream on Madison Run Fire Road to the Furnace Mountain Trail. Turn left on the Furnace Mountain Trail and then cross Madison Run. Go briefly downstream, turn left, and start the steep climb up the western side of Furnace Mountain, coming to a gap and a trail junction at mile 8.2.

Make the side trip to the summit of Furnace Mountain by turning left and ascending half a mile to the summit and an outcrop. Look across at Austin Mountain. Directly below you is Madison Run.

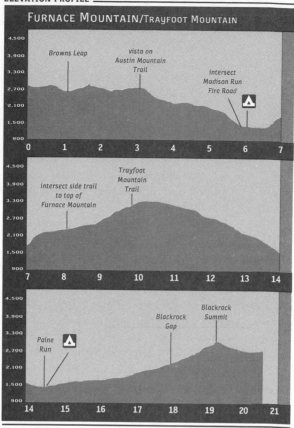

FURNACE MOUNTAIN/TRAYFOOT MOUNTAIN

Leave the gap and walk along the ridge through a forest of pine and mountain laurel. Start climbing, making two sharp turns: first right and then left. Enter a talus slope on the northern flank of Trayfoot Mountain and come to Trayfoot Mountain Trail at mile 10.

Turn right on the old roadbed of the Trayfoot Mountain Trail, reaching the ridge's crest at mile 10.2. The official peak is a few hundred feet down the road to the left. When you turn right at the ridge's crest, views open up as the footpath undulates along the crest. Begin a long descent and be glad you are going down instead of up.

Switchback to the left into Lefthand Hollow at mile 13.8 and then make another switchback to the right, coming to Paine Run at mile 14.4. Lower Lefthand Hollow and the first mile of Paine Run have several suitable campsites. This is your second night's destination.

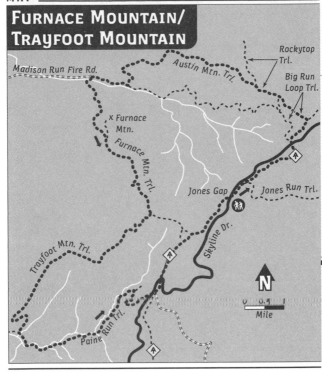

🚶 DAY 3 Start day three on the Paine Run Trail. At mile 14.6 of your loop hike, rock hop Paine Run, an exceptionally attractive stream with clear water tumbling over tan rocks. Leave Paine Run at mile 15.3 and enter a pine–mountain laurel woodland. The trail begins a pattern, climbing moderately, briefly dipping as it crosses one of several feeder streams, rising, and finally resuming its moderate grade. Some of these tributary streams will be dry at certain times of the year. Intermittent views of Horsehead and Trayfoot Mountains open up to your left.

As Paine Run Hollow narrows, the forest slowly changes character from open pine to lush hardwood. When the tree canopy closes overhead, Blackrock Springs is not far away. At mile 17.1 the road switchbacks sharply to the right. Look for a footpath to your left that leads to the springs and a resort site that operated in one form or another for more than a century. There may be a few fallen trees in the way but work around them, and soon you'll come to building foundations, flat spots, and springs.

Return to the Paine Run Trail and turn left. Climb onto a dry ridge and reach Blackrock Gap at

mile 18.1. Cross Skyline Drive and turn left on the
AT. Your northbound route soon takes you back
across Skyline Drive. Ascend past the side trail to
Blackrock Hut at mile 18.8.

Stay on the AT and come to Blackrock Summit
at mile 19.4. Here you can see the terrain you've
covered: Austin Mountain, Furnace Mountain,
Trayfoot Mountain, Madison Run, and Paine Run.
Continue north on the AT, passing the Trayfoot
Mountain Trail, and cross Skyline Drive once more
before completing your loop at the Jones Run parking area (mile 20.6).

DIRECTIONS: From the Rockfish Gap entrance station,
drive north on Skyline Drive for 21.3 miles to the Jones Run
parking area (mile 83.3), which will be on your right.

Moormans River

SCENERY: ☆ ☆ ☆ ☆
TRAIL CONDITION: ☆ ☆ ☆
CHILDREN: ☆ ☆
DIFFICULTY: ☆ ☆
SOLITUDE: ☆ ☆ ☆ ☆
DISTANCE: *Day 1, 5.4 miles; Day 2, 5.3 miles; Day 3, 7.4 miles*
HIKING TIME: *3:30, 3:30, 4:45 hours*
OUTSTANDING FEATURES: *views, waterfalls, swimming holes, trout fishing, old
homesites*

THIS LOOP TAKES YOU ALONG THE CREST *of the Blue Ridge into
the upper Moormans River watershed and back around to the high
country. Ply the Appalachian Trail (AT) and savor some views before
entering the North Fork of the Moormans River valley where effects
of a 1995 flood still show. Camp in the vicinity of Big Branch Falls
before heading to the South Fork of the Moormans River valley,
where deep pools and waterfalls await. The next day, camp in the
upper part of the valley before rejoining the AT and cruising the high
country on the park's rocky spine. Travel distances are divided fairly
evenly, but your last day is the longest when your pack will be light-
est. In late spring and summer, bring a fishing rod and swimming
trunks. Be apprised that this trip entails several river crossings. If the
rivers are at or near flood stage, save this loop for another time.*

 ♯♯ DAY 1 Start your loop at the Riprap parking
area and follow the Riprap Trail a few feet to meet the
AT. Head north on the AT and climb through stand-

ing dead trees, victims of gypsy moths and/or fire to reach a junction at 0.5 miles. The Riprap Trail heads to the left (see the Chimney Rock hike description if you want to take a side trip, p.48), otherwise continue forward along the AT, which offers views of Pasture Fence Mountain to your right. Descend to cross Skyline Drive at mile 1.2. The AT circles around the eastern side of a knob, passing through a forest of slender striped maples. Draw near Skyline Drive in a gap then ascend among more young trees. Undulate along the ridgecrest to finally descend among rocky woods, making Blackrock Gap at mile 3. Turn right here, following the yellow-blazed North Fork Moormans River Fire Road. Shortly cross a feeder stream of the river that the trail begins to parallel, reaching a gate at mile 4.1. Leave the park and reach a junction at 4.4 miles. Turn right and cross the North Fork of the Moormans River on rocks. Look for secretive brook trout in the pool above the crossing. Turn right at a second junction after passing a ramshackle hunter's camp. Cross the river again at mile 4.6 in a deep and thick forest.

A yellow gate and Little Gale Branch mark your reentry into the park at mile 5.1. Your route past the gate now officially becomes the North Fork Moormans River Trail. Begin looking for a campsite in the flats along both sides of the river in the next mile or so. You must be at least a quarter mile inside the park boundary to legally camp.

🐾 DAY 2 Start day two by looking for the remnants of mudslides from the 1995 flood. Although the once-barren slopes are slowly becoming reforested, the old roadbed of the trail along with a metal bridge was washed out.

Cross Big Branch at mile 6.6. Here, the bouldery stream cascades toward the North Fork on your left. A side trail leads upstream 0.1 mile to Big Branch Falls. Keep forward beyond Big Branch, nearing the North Fork, then head away onto the washed out roadbed. Look for huge boulders in the river and bluffs overlooking it. More mudslides are evident as well.

Cross the North Fork at mile 7.4, and stay close to the river, nearing rock slabs that provide quick access to the water. At mile 8, cross the river twice in succession, working around a beautiful multicolored bluff. The valley begins to widen as the trail soon leaves the park. Keep forward on the roadbed, passing

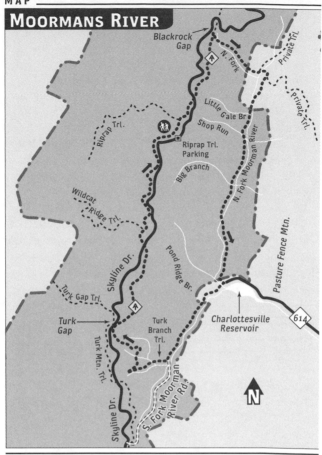

MOORMANS RIVER

Blackrock Gap

N. Fork

Riprap Trl.

Little Gale Br

Shop Run

Private Trl.

Private Trl.

N. Fork Moorman River

Riprap Trl. Parking

Big Branch

Wildcat Ridge Trl.

Pond Ridge Br.

Skyline Dr.

Pasture Fence Mtn.

Turk Gap Trl.

Charlottesville Reservoir

614

Turk Gap

Turk Branch Trl.

Turk Mtn. Trl.

Skyline Dr.

S. Fork Moorman River Rd.

N

a signboard and parking area. Follow an access road to reach VA 614 at mile 8.6. As VA 614 climbs left, you should turn right on the South Fork Moormans River Fire Road at a sign stating "Fire Road, Do Not Block." A concrete trail post marks the turn. Shortly cross the North Fork one final time, and look left into the Charlottesville Reservoir. Skirt around a metal gate, resuming a southbound course, climbing to rock hop the South Fork at mile 9.5. This is an ultra attractive mountain stream in a heavily wooded valley. At mile 10, look on trail left for a standing chimney of a former homestead. Think of the time spent in front of that hearth during days gone by. Ahead, look for a huge rock outcrop to the left and a deep pool below a cascade. A deeper pool and bigger waterfall is just upstream of this point, beckoning weary feet and sweaty bodies.

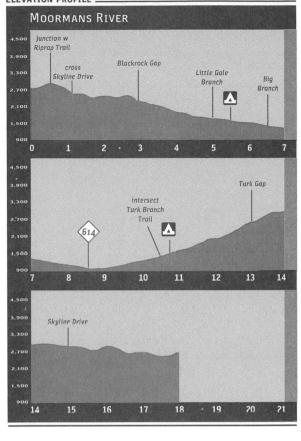

MOORMANS RIVER

Stay right as an old road leads left. Look for the rock foundation and an old stone fence marking a homesite. Step over the South Fork at mile 10.5. Soon, fully reenter the park past a gate. (The park has been on the far side of the river for some distance.) Intersect the Turk Gap Trail at mile 10.7. Piled stones and leveled land suggest a former homesite to the right of the trail, which meets the South Fork Moormans River Fire Road. A USGS survey marker has been embedded into a boulder at the junction. Begin to look for a campsite either up Turk Branch hollow to your right or ahead on South Fork Moormans River, which has flats up the fire road. Remember that you must be at least a quarter mile inside the park's boundary to camp.

🏃 DAY 3 Start day three by turning up the Turk Branch Trail. Pass the old homesite on your right to cross Turk Branch at mile 11.2. Notice the stonework used to level the old roadbed. A small cascade drops above the Turk Branch crossing. Ascend a feeder branch of Turk Branch, crossing the feeder branch twice near more stonework. Curve uphill back to Turk Branch, stepping over its upper reaches at mile 11.9. Keep ascending in an open canopied pine forest mixed with mountain laurel to near Skyline Drive at mile 12.8. The Turk Branch Trail parallels the drive north to reach Turk Gap at mile 13.1. Keep forward across the Turk Gap parking area to intersect the AT. Head northbound on the AT, ascending away from Turk Gap in oak woods with a rock and brush under-story. Most rocks have been cleared from the trail, which levels out at mile 13.7 and gains the crest of the ridge. Enjoy the mostly level ramble, letting your legs carry you forward with your senses absorbing the sights, sounds, and smells of nature. The forest is low slung and piney at a high point before drifting down-ward to cross Skyline Drive at mile 15. Curve downhill through burned woods—blackened tree trunks and an evenly aged understory are evidence of a past fire. Keep forward through the Wildcat Ridge Trail junc-tion at mile 15.3. A sporadically open canopy can make this trail hot in the afternoon. A sparse pine forest at mile 16 allows far-reaching views to the west.

The AT crosses over to the eastern side of the ridge among tree skeletons standing over younger live trees. With views now to the east, work around a knob back to the west side of the ridge. Rocks Mountain is visible westward through the trees by mile 17. The AT traverses a scree slope at mile 17.5, while nearby Skyline Drive seems to stand on end. Curve around the ridgeline to the right and climb, intersecting the Riprap Trail at mile 18.1. Turn right and walk just a few feet to the Riprap parking area, completing the loop.

DIRECTIONS: From Rockfish Gap entrance station, head north on Skyline Drive for 14.6 miles to Riprap parking area, mile 90, on your left.

Index